Sniffly Sandborn
in
A Trip to the Hospital

By Denise Trager and Mary Ellen Panaccione
Artwork by Greg Pugh   Text by Stephen Greco

Copyright 2015

SONGS

Sniffly Sandborn in a Trip to the Hospital features hit songs that you can listen to as you read along!

Visit www.HuggableMelodies.com/Sandborn to listen to the songs on any pages with a song button like this one:

CHARACTERS

Poindexter

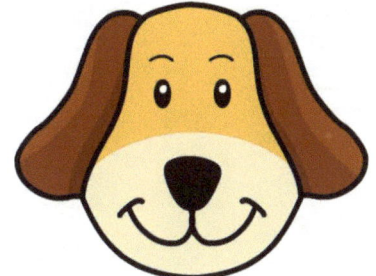

Sandborn

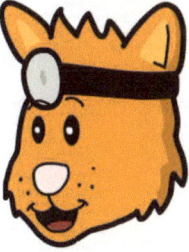

Dr. Seva - pediatrician

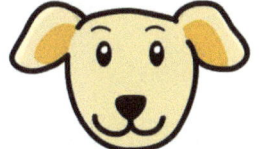

Drysdale

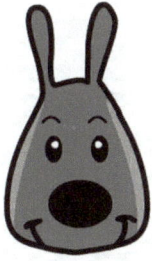

Bonky

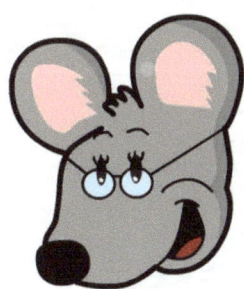

Dr. Tso - surgeon

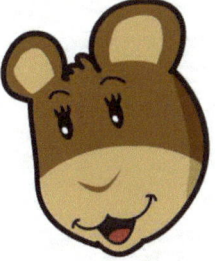

Dr. Yashen - anesthesiologist

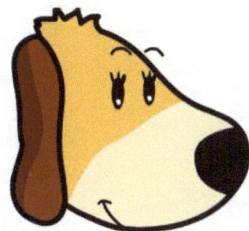

Sandborn's mom

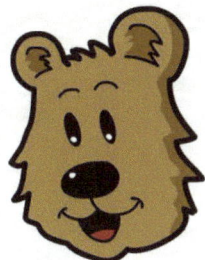

Nurse Rodney

Sandborn had been excited for weeks about his upcoming birthday party! It was going to take place on Saturday—just five days away! At school on Monday, Sandborn's friends were all talking about the party.
"Can't wait!" said Poindexter.
"It's going to be so much fun!" said Drysdale.

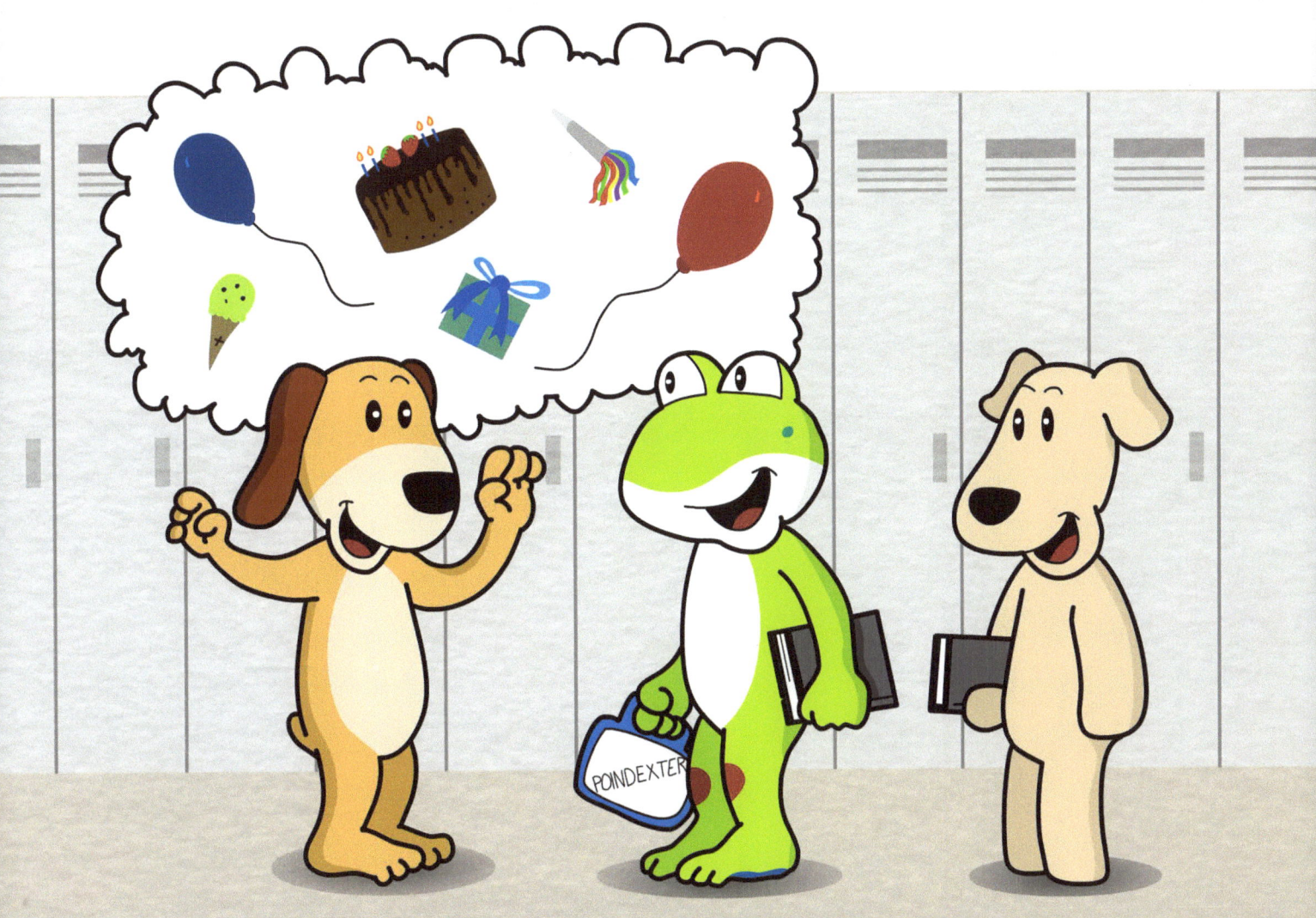

Even Bonky was excited. He was a new friend that Sandborn made after Poindexter showed everybody how nice Bonky could be, now that he wasn't a bully anymore.

"Are you going to have a cake?" asked Bonky.

"Of course," said Sandborn. "Mom is making my favorite — chocolate with strawberries"

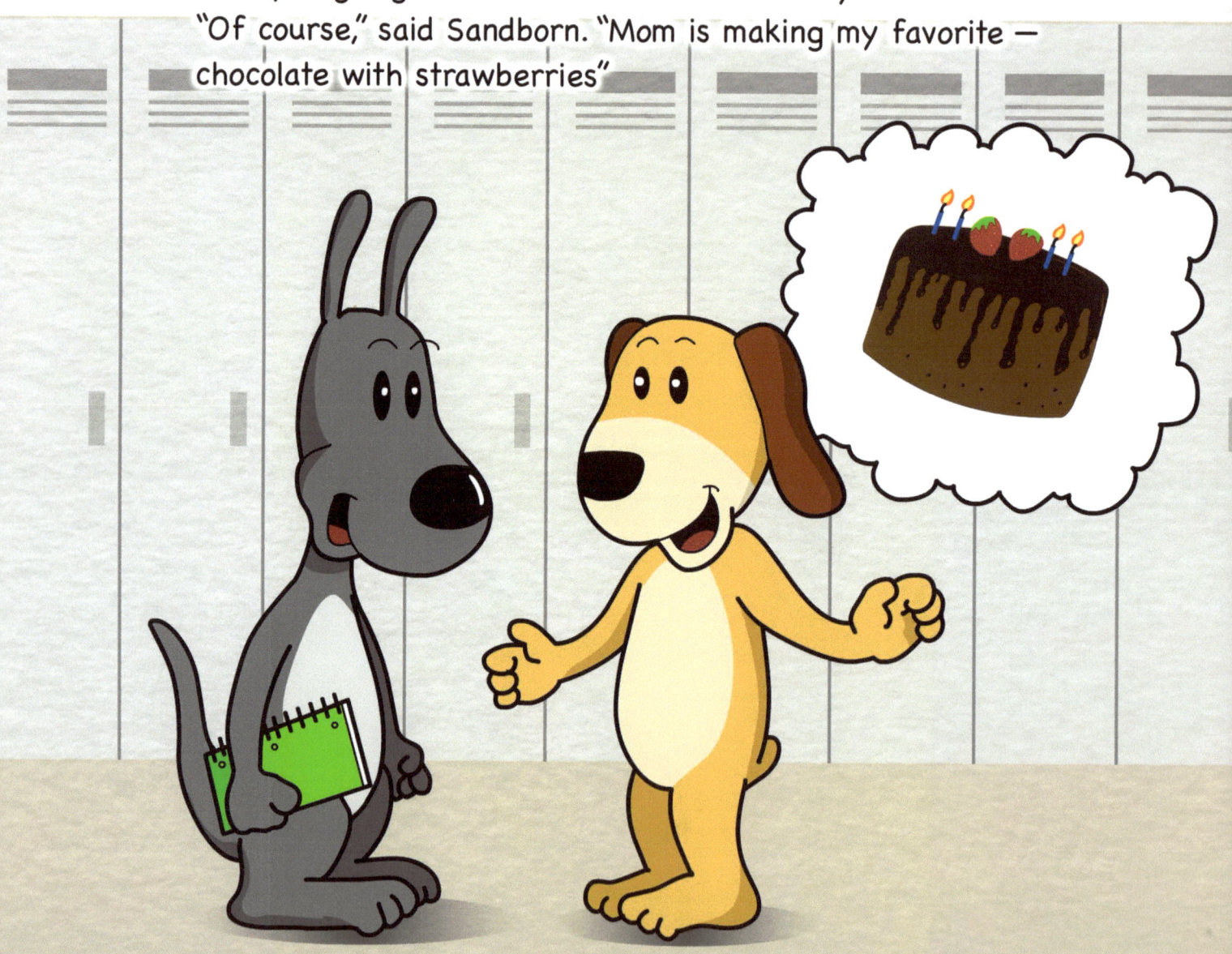

But, earlier that morning, Sandborn felt a familiar tickle in his throat that meant a sore throat might be coming.

"Uh-oh," he thought. He had been getting so many sore throats and colds that some kids called him "Sniffly Sandborn" - not the nicest nickname in the world!

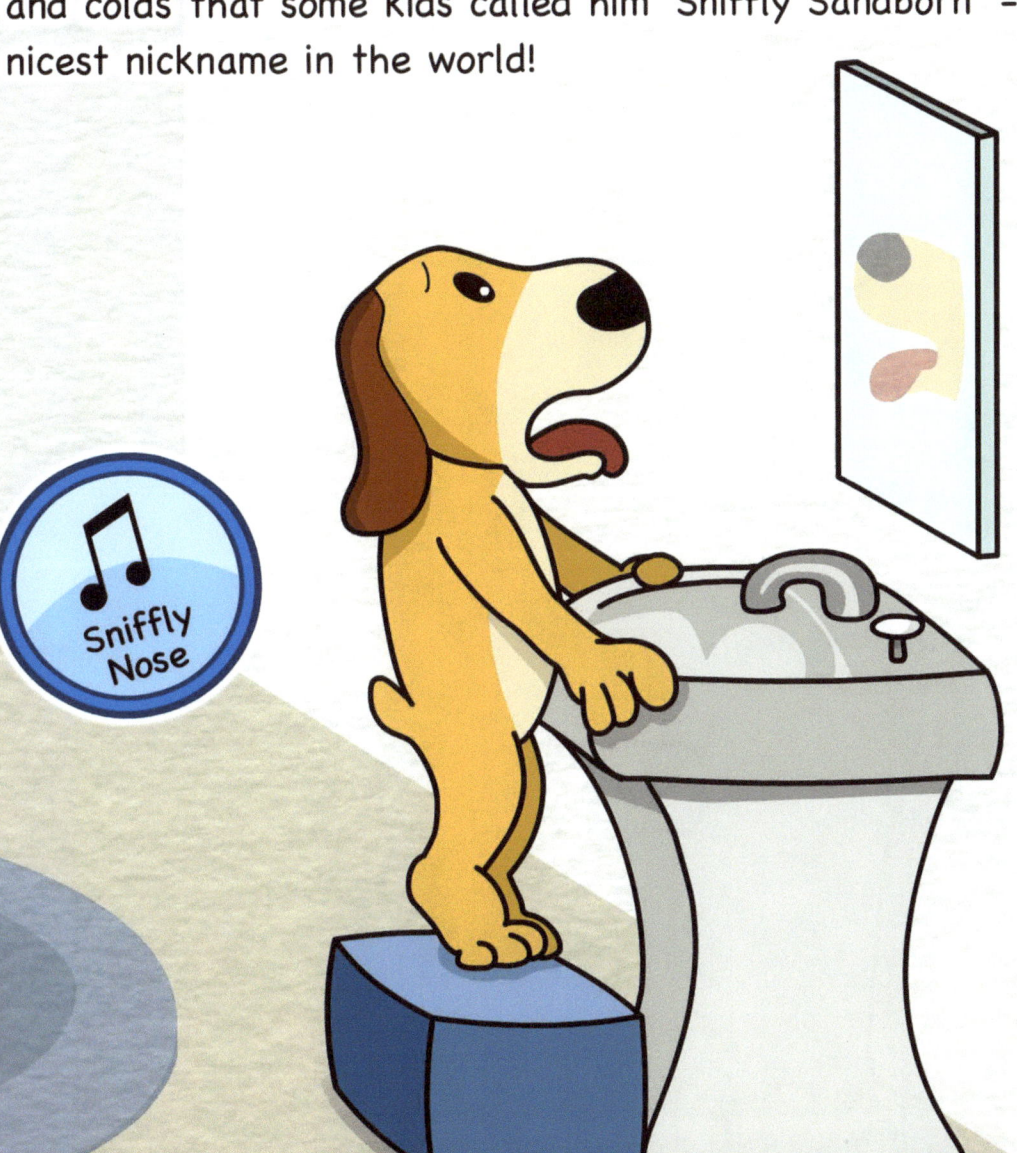

Sure enough, by lunchtime Sandborn felt a lump in his throat when he swallowed, and the inside of his ears ached. Sandborn's teacher noticed him sniffling, so she sent him to the school nurse.
The nurse took one look at Sandborn's throat and said, "Oh, yes, I can see it's red." She also took his temperature. "A slight fever," she said. "I'd better send you home."

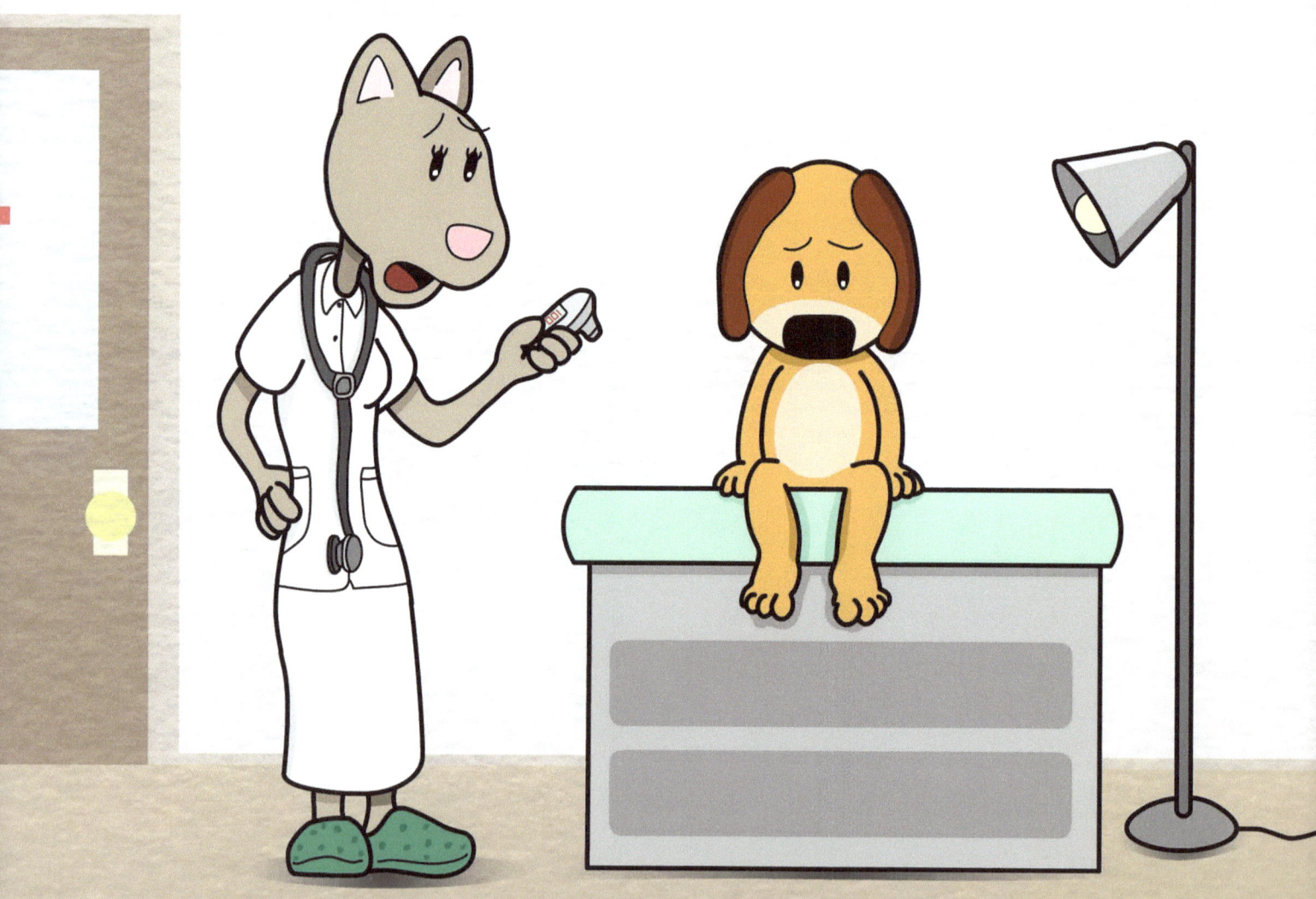

Sandborn's mom drove him home from school and put him straight to bed. She brought Sandborn some juice to drink, his favorite stuffed animal, and a fresh box of tissues.

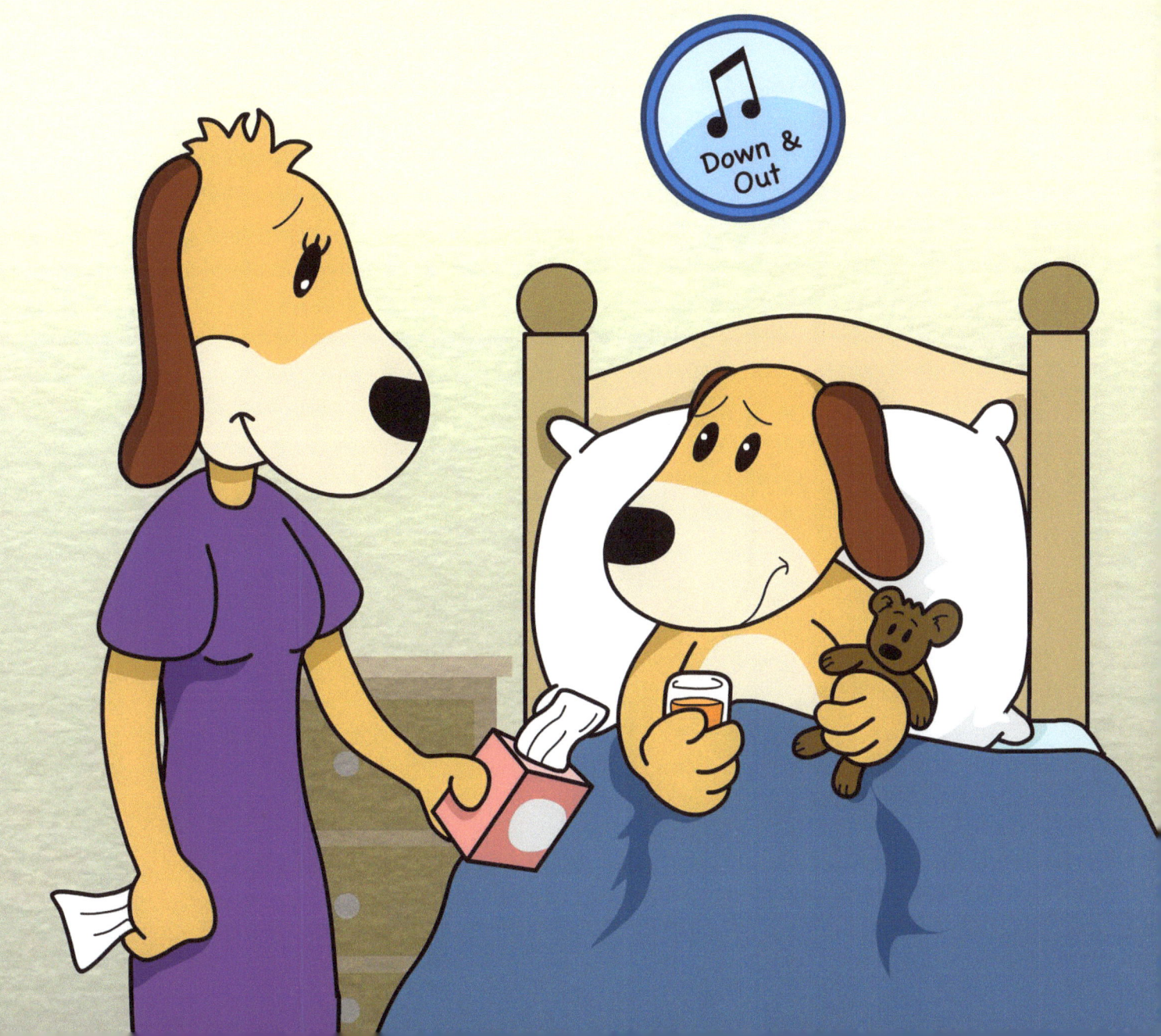

The next morning, Sandborn still had the sniffles and a fever, so his mom called the doctor. "You'd better bring him in," said Dr. Seva. As Sandborn and his mom drove to the doctor's office, he felt miserable. Not only was he sniffling, but his throat and ears hurt, too. "Mom, I hope I am better by Saturday."
"I hope so too, sweetie."
Slumped in his seat, Sandborn was quiet the rest of the way.

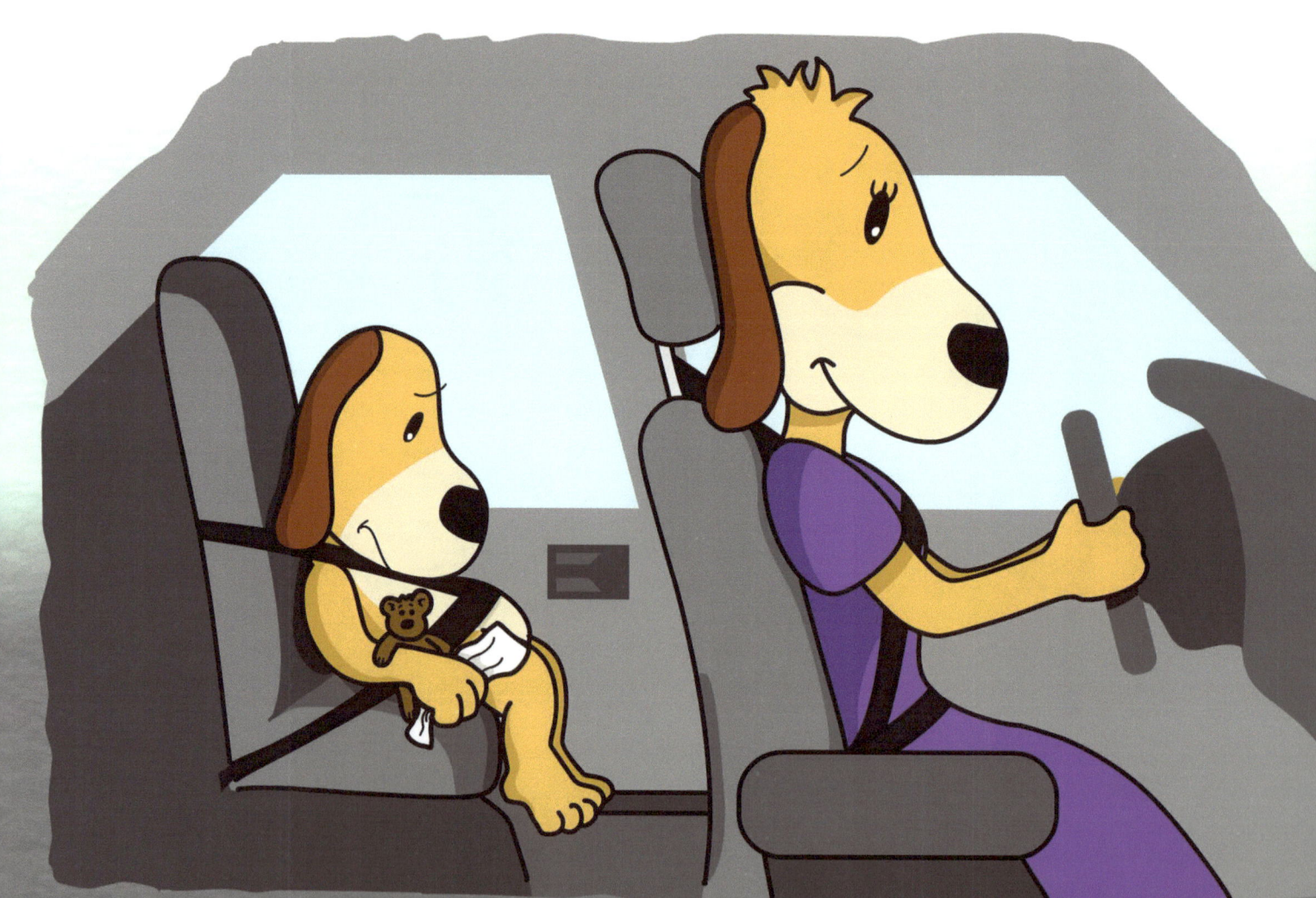

Dr. Seva examined Sandborn carefully, explaining what he was doing and telling him the names of the instruments he was using. With his ophthalmoscope he looked at Sandborn's eyes. With his otoscope he looked at Sandborn's nose and ears. With a simple tongue depressor he looked in his throat. Very carefully Dr. Seva listened to Sandborn's heart and lungs with his stethoscope, and with a thermometer he took his temperature.

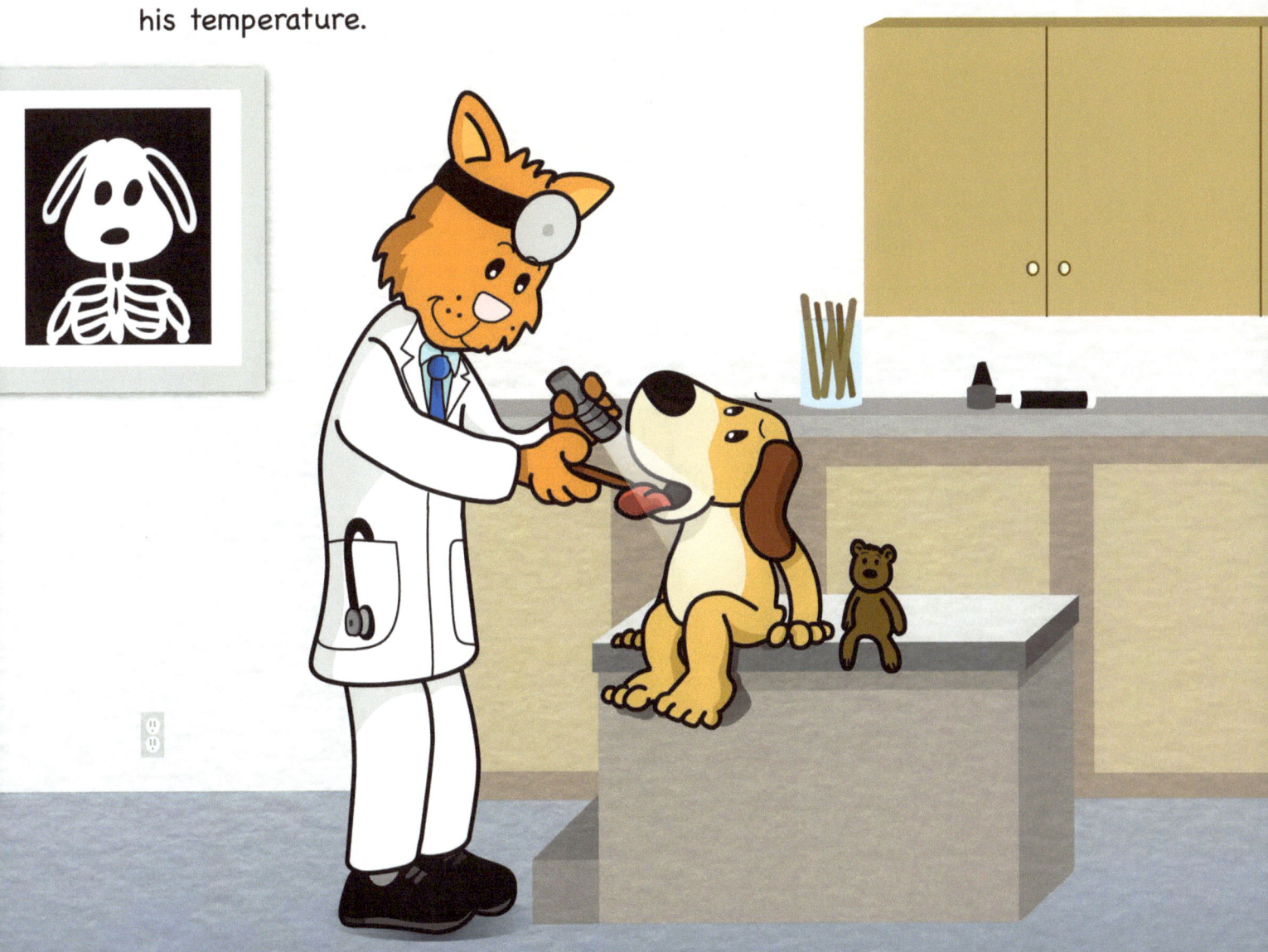

"I'm concerned that he's getting so many of these sore throats,"
said Dr. Seva to Sandborn's mom. "Remember when I said he might
need to have his tonsils and adenoids out?" His mom nodded. "Well,"
said the doctor gently, "I think now is the time for the operation."
"**Operation**?", said Sandborn. "What's an operation? And will it be
over by Saturday?"
"I'll explain everything to you in a little bit," said Dr. Seva. "But
right now I need to check your lungs.

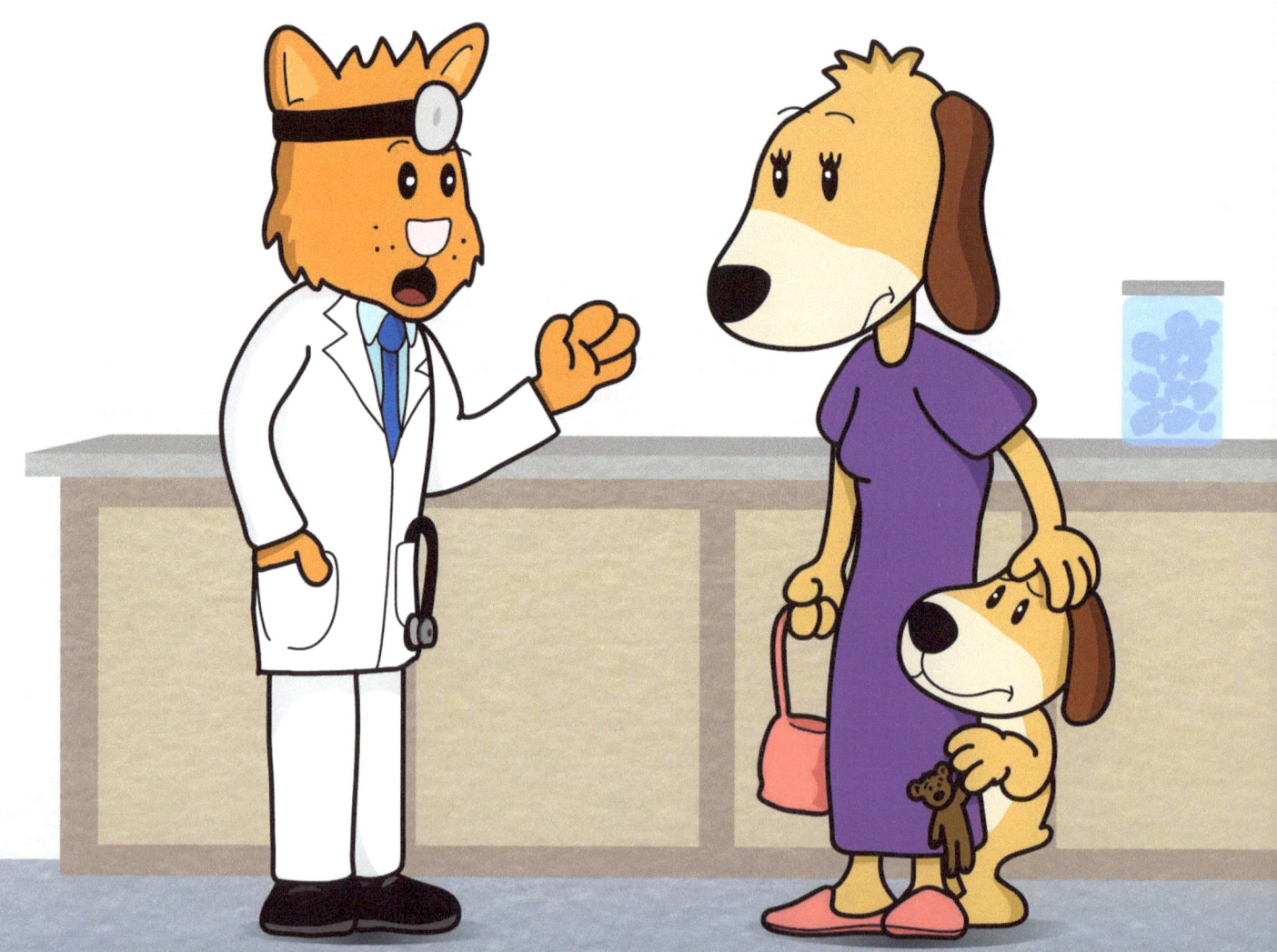

"How do you check my lungs?" said Sandborn.

"With an x-ray machine and pictures", said the doctor. "They show us what is going on inside your body."

Dr. Seva took Sandborn and his mom down the hallway and into a special room where a technician stood Sandborn in front of a big machine. The technician explained they were going to take a picture of his lungs.

In a few seconds it was all over! And Sandborn didn't feel a thing!

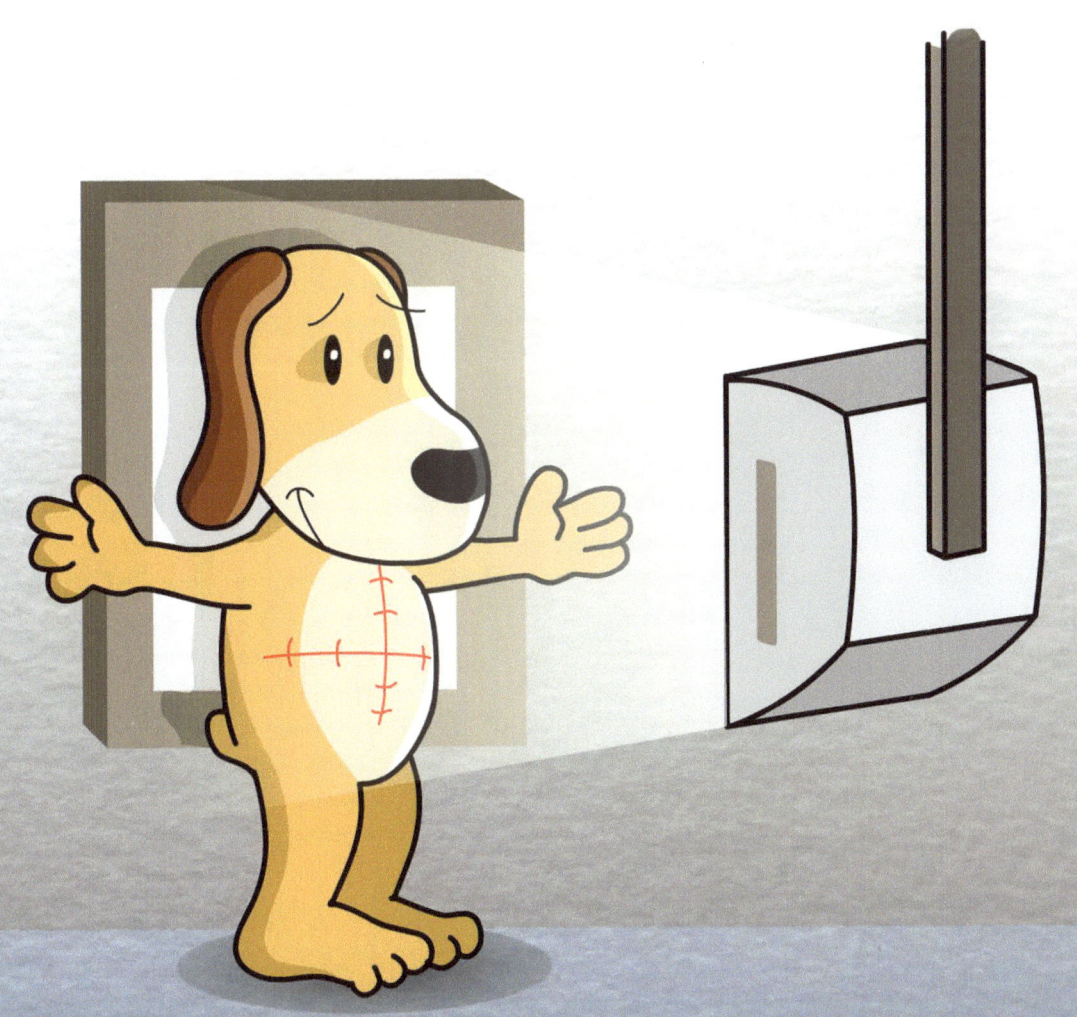

Back in the doctor's office, Dr. Seva said that Sandborn's lungs looked fine -- But he would definitely need the operation to remove his tonsils and adenoids.

"What are tonsils, anyway, and what are ade... ade...," said Sandborn. "Adenoids," said Dr. Seva, who explained with the help of a diagram hanging on the wall. "They're organs—part of the body's immune system which helps your body fight infection. Tonsils are in the back of your throat, and adenoids are right behind your nose. Usually, they help detect bad bacteria. But sometimes they get infected too much, like yours, and need to come out."

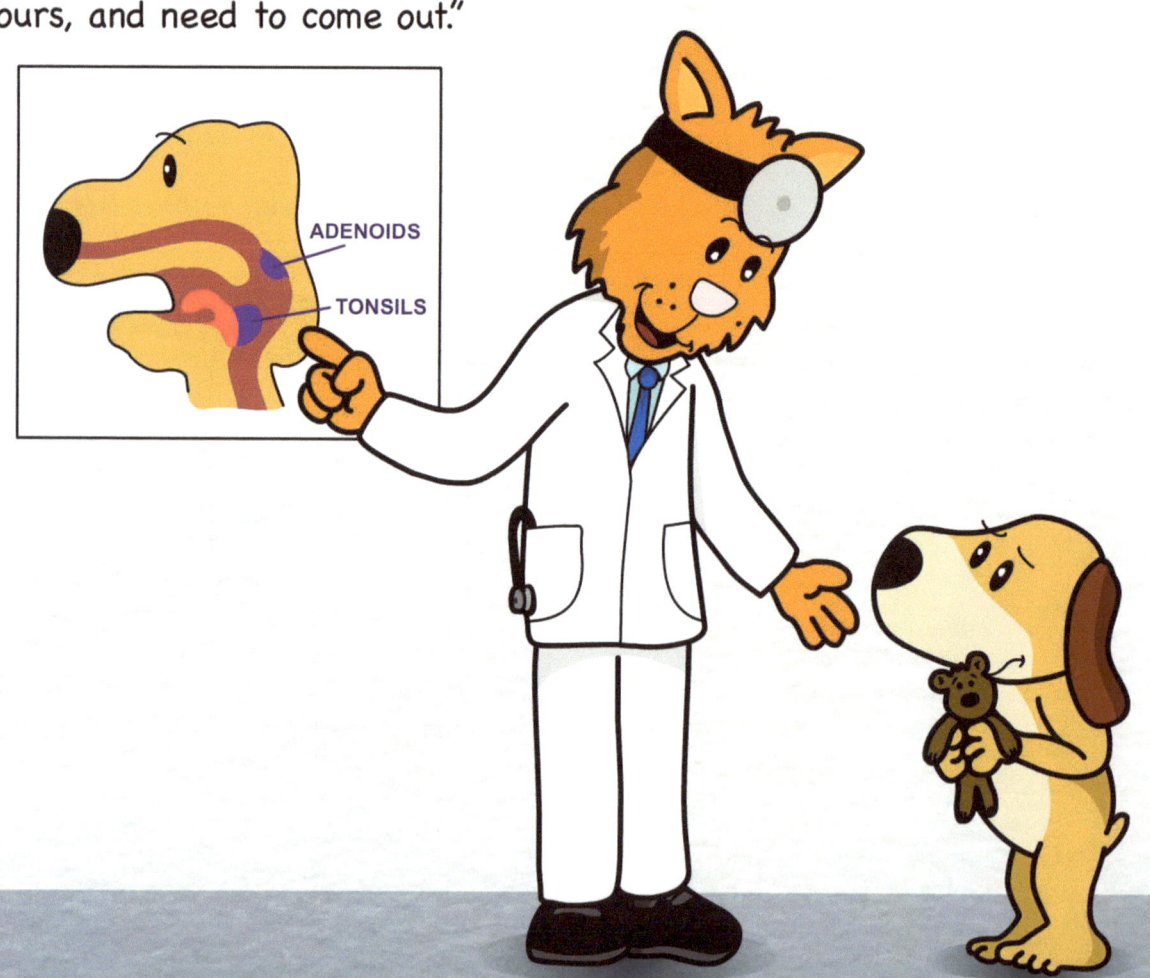

ADENOIDS

TONSILS

"How do you get them out?" Sandborn asked.

"A surgeon makes a little snip and removes them." said Dr. Seva. "It's very simple."

"Whats a surgeon?" he asked.

"A surgeon is a doctor who knows how to make a tiny cut that heals quickly."

"A tiny cut?!" Will it hurt?"

"Not at all! Another doctor called an anesthesiologist will help you go to sleep before the operation. And the best part is that afterwards you won't have so many sore throats or be so sniffly!"

The doctor explained that before the operation they had to eliminate Sandborn's throat infection and fever. That would take a few days, he said, so he scheduled the operation for Friday morning.

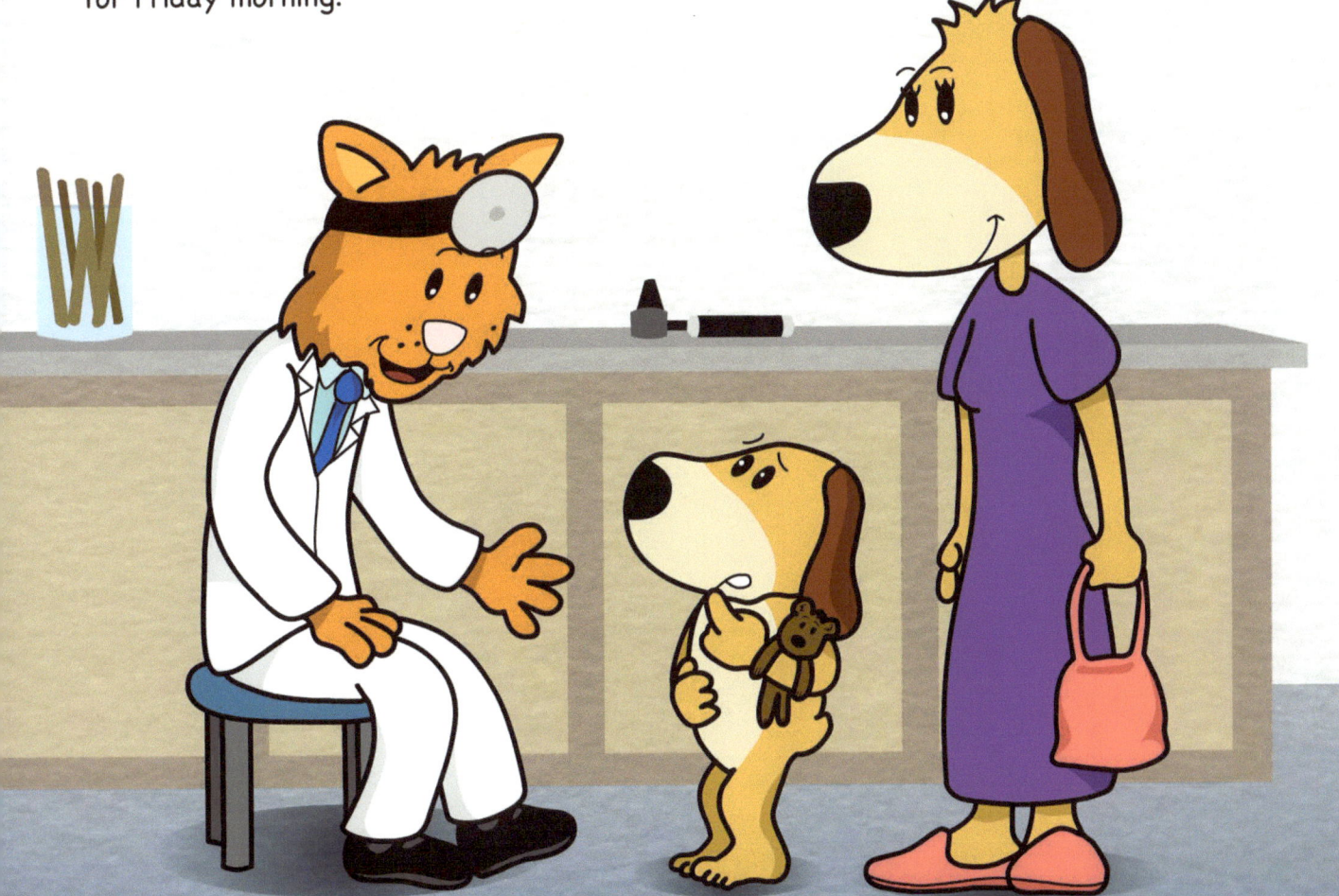

Sandborn was quiet almost all the way home from the doctor's office. Then, as they pulled into the driveway, he brought up the issue that was on his mind.

"Mom, since my operation is on Friday, we can still have the party on Saturday, right?"

Sandborn's mom made a frowny little smile. "Oh, sweetie, I don't know," she said. "Your health is the most important thing right now, isn't it?"

"The doctor said it was only a little snip...," said Sandborn.

His mom squeezed his arm gently.

"Well, I suppose we might be able to do it...," she said. "We'll just have to see what the doctor says."

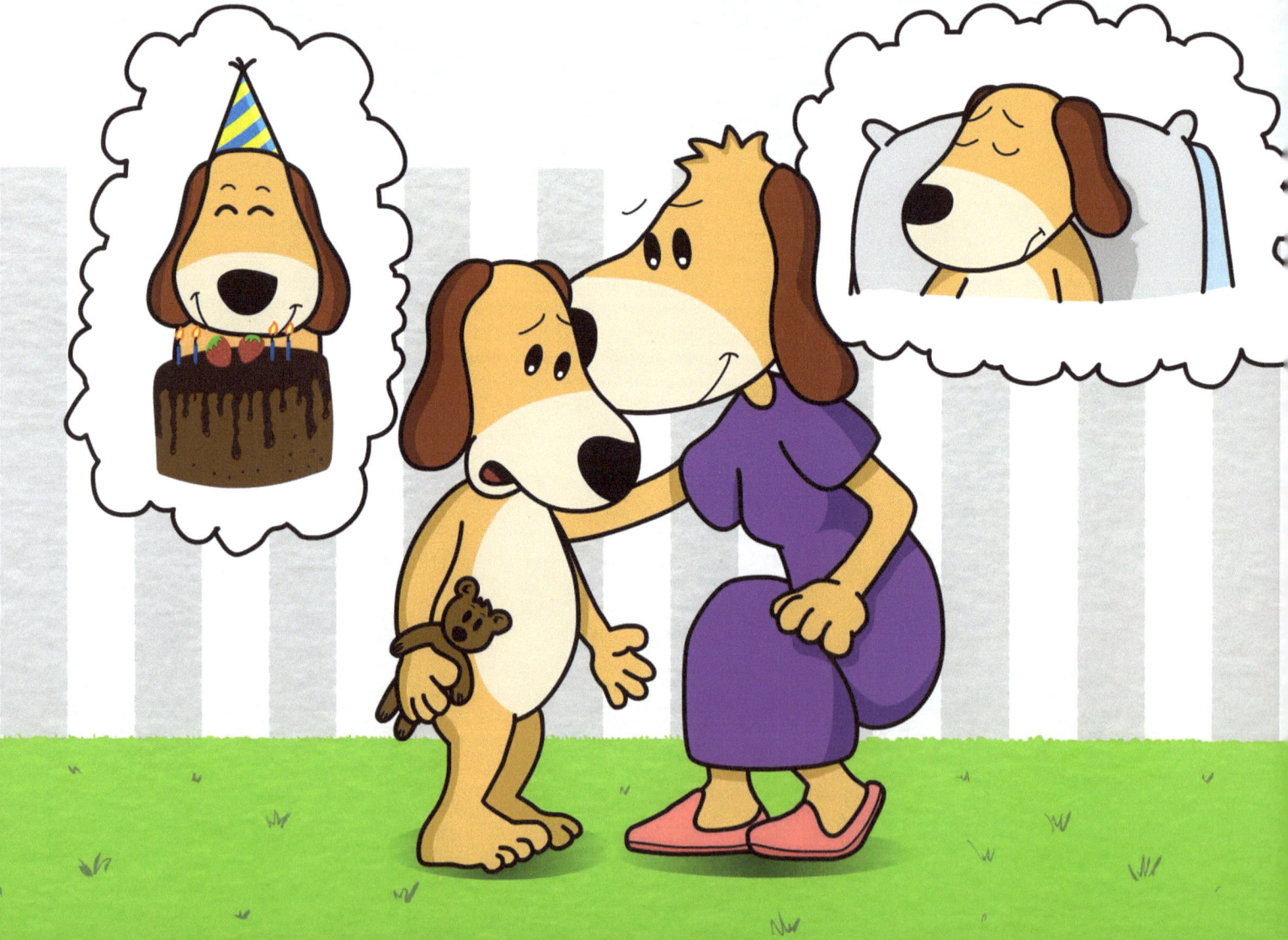

Over the next few days, Sandborn eagerly took the medicine that Dr. Seva prescribed. He was determined to be a good patient, so the fever would go away and the operation could take place on schedule — which would mean that his birthday party could take place, on Saturday, as planned.

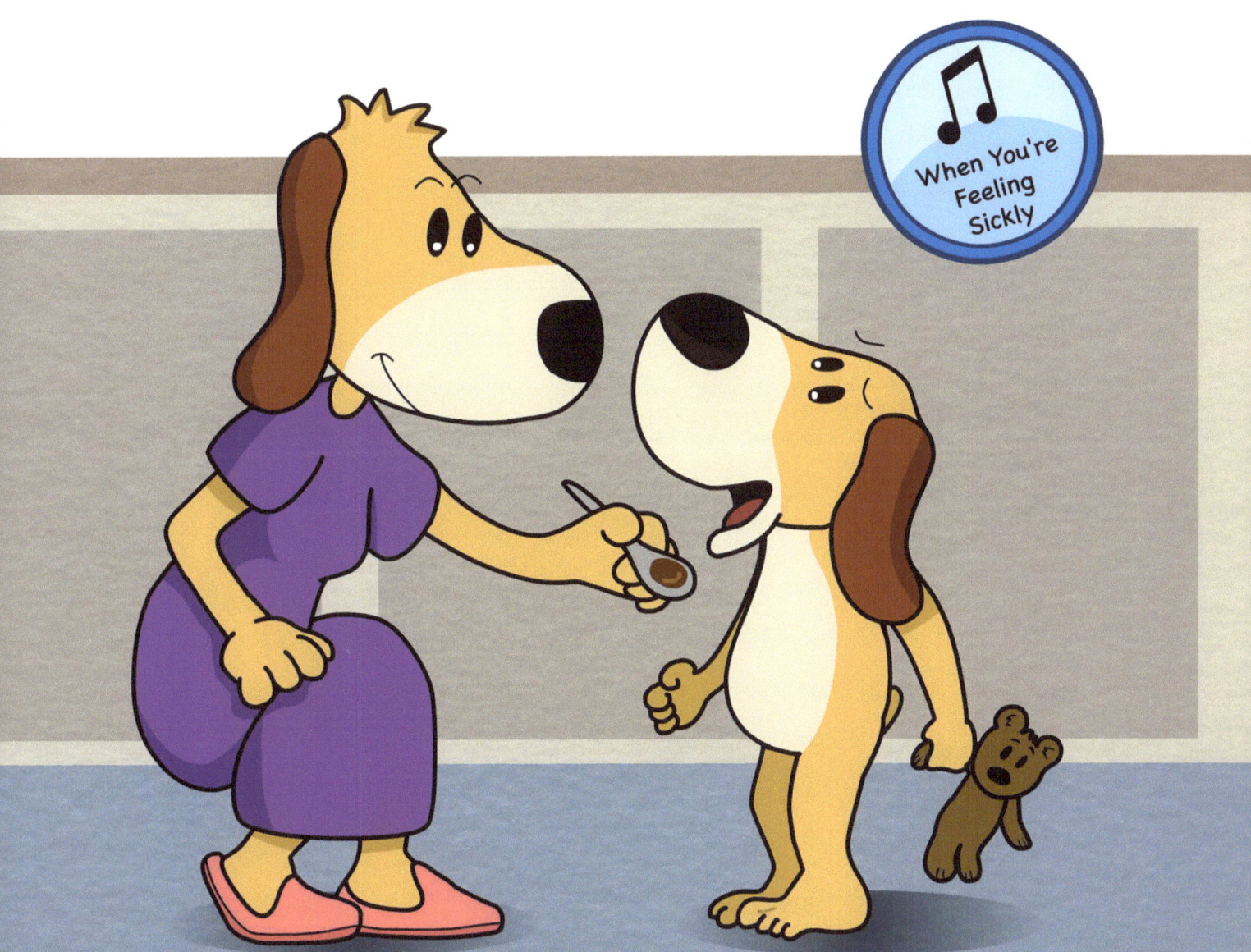

When You're Feeling Sickly

And sure enough, by Thursday morning the fever was gone. But that day at school, Sandborn was nervous about the next day's operation, and he mentioned this to Bonky and Poindexter. They told him not to worry. They said they both knew friends who'd had their tonsils and adenoids out, and it was no big deal.

"You get to eat lots of ice cream afterward," said Poindexter.

"Yeah, but I might not be having my birthday party," said Sandborn. "It's supposed to be on Saturday, but Mom says I might not be out of the hospital."

"Hmm," said Bonky. "Well, I'm sure we can figure out how to have another party."

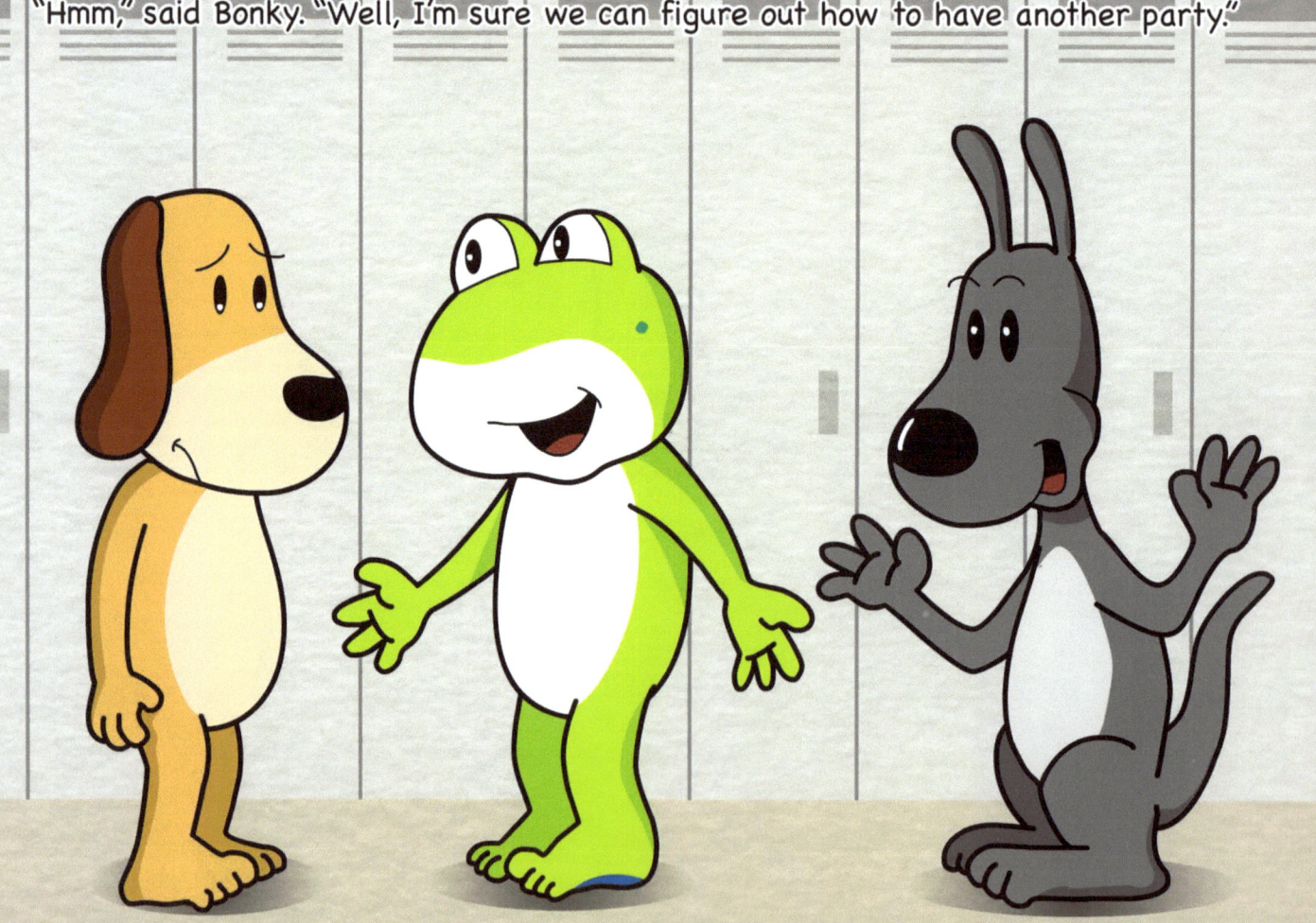

That night, Sandborn's mom reminded him there was no snacking after supper.
Dr. Seva had said that this was an important part of getting ready for an
operation.

And very early Friday morning, around 7 they drove to the hospital and
checked in. Sandborn and his mom met Nurse Rodney who took them to a room
where Sandborn put on a hospital gown and got into bed.

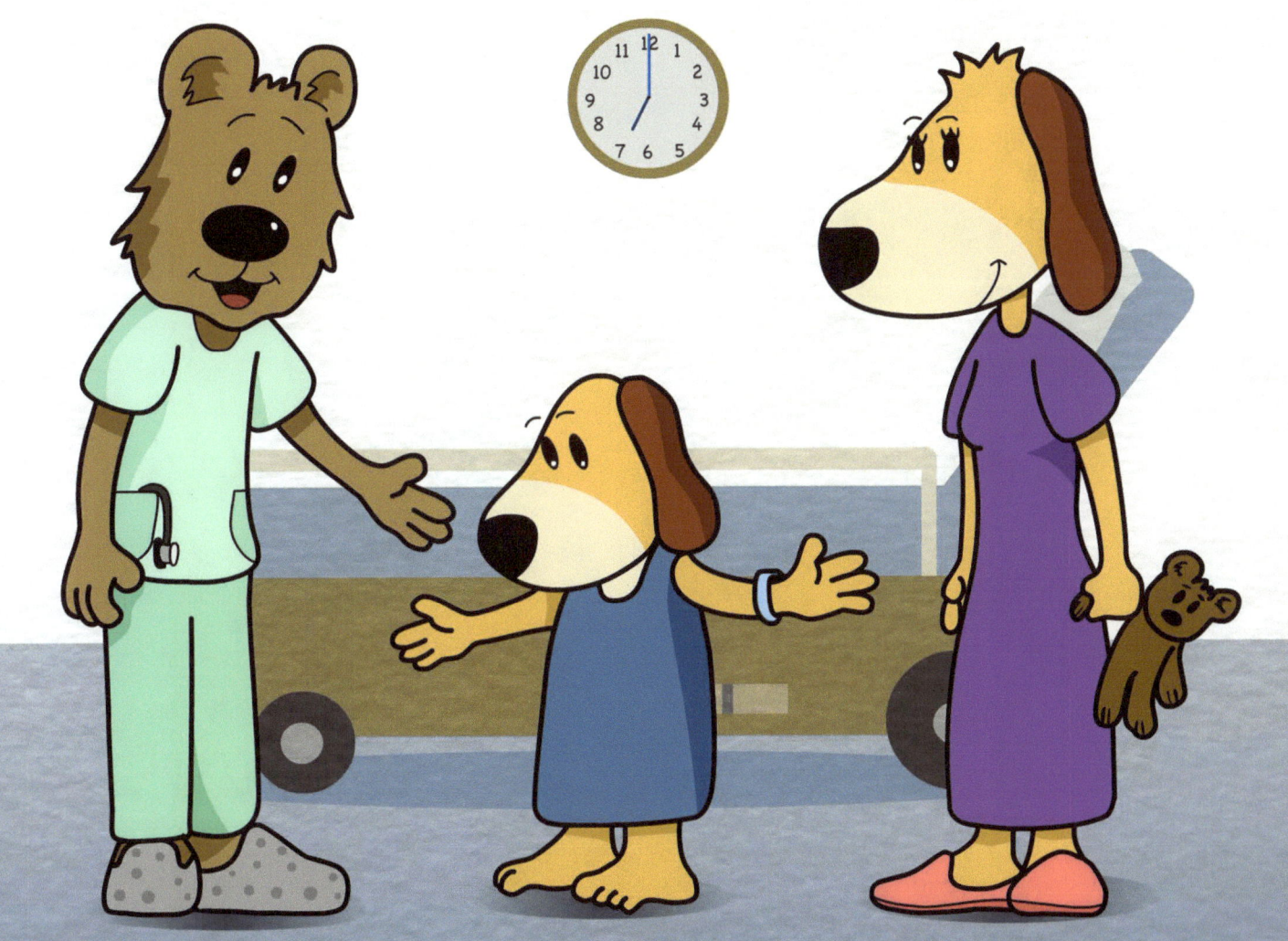

"Will I be able to go home tonight?" asked Sandborn.
"I hope so, but we will have to check with your doctor. You may have to stay a night or two if you develop any minor complications."
"If you do stay, we'll have fun!" said mom. "We'll play games and eat ice cream!"

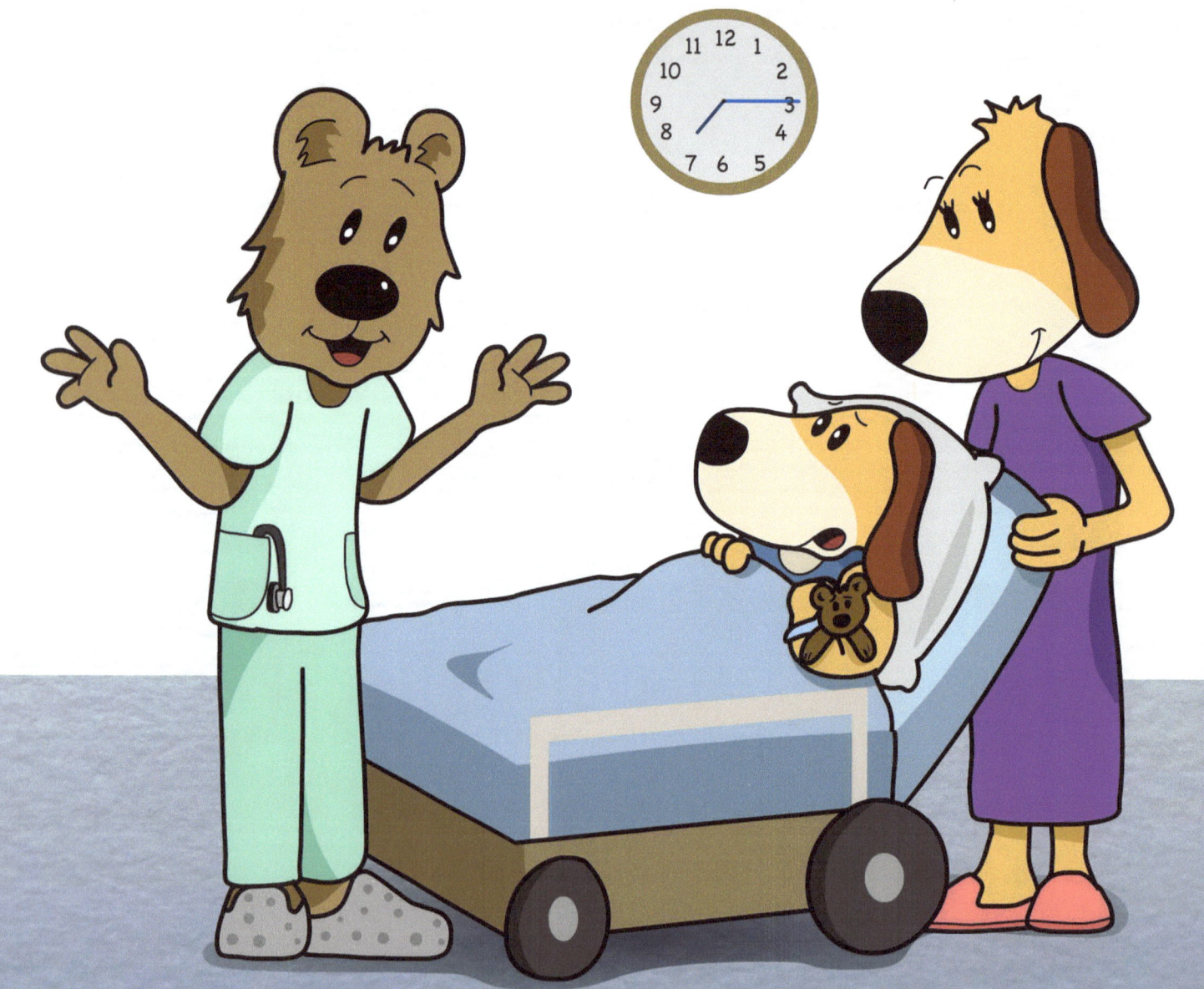

Then everything got very busy! At 8, a nice doctor came in and introduced herself as the anesthesiologist, Dr. Yashen. She explained that in a little while, in the operating room, she was going to put Sandborn to sleep and that it wouldn't hurt a bit. She examined Sandborn and asked a few questions about how he was feeling. Then she said, "See you soon, Sandborn!"

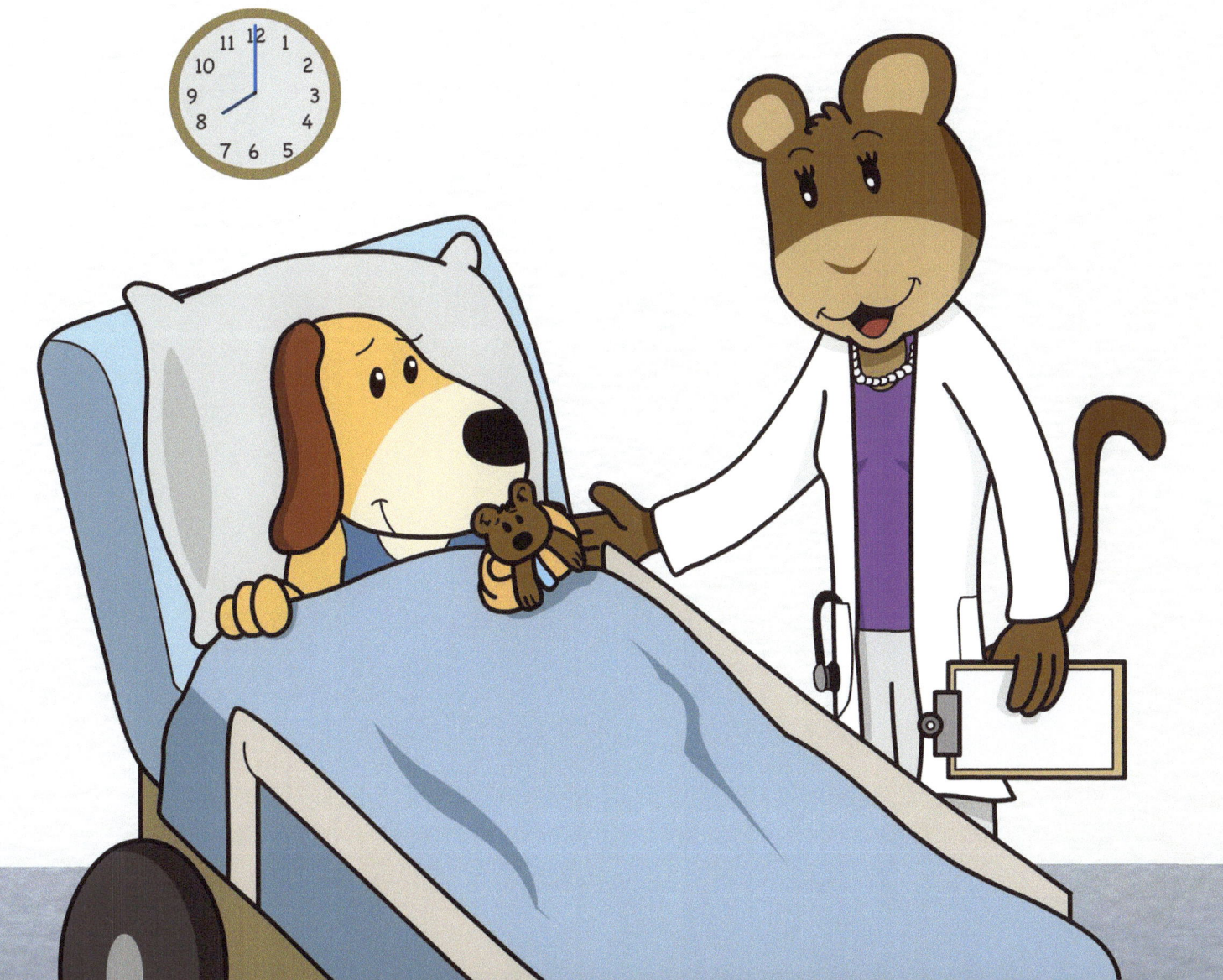

At 9, Nurse Rodney came to the room with a bed on wheels - a gurney, he called it - and helped Sandborn get onto it. He prepared Sandborn for anesthesia by putting a small catheter with a needle into a vein in his arm. The needle didn't hurt because Nurse Rodney had something special to rub on Sandborn's arm first. Once the catheter was in the right place, Nurse Rodney took the needle out and left the catheter in the vein. Then he connected the catheter to the IV bag.

They were all off to the operating room....down the corridors of the hospital, up in and elevator, and finally through two sets of double doors. Nurse Rodney told Sandborn that his mom could go into the operating room with him and stay until he was asleep. And then, during the operation, she would be right outside the door.

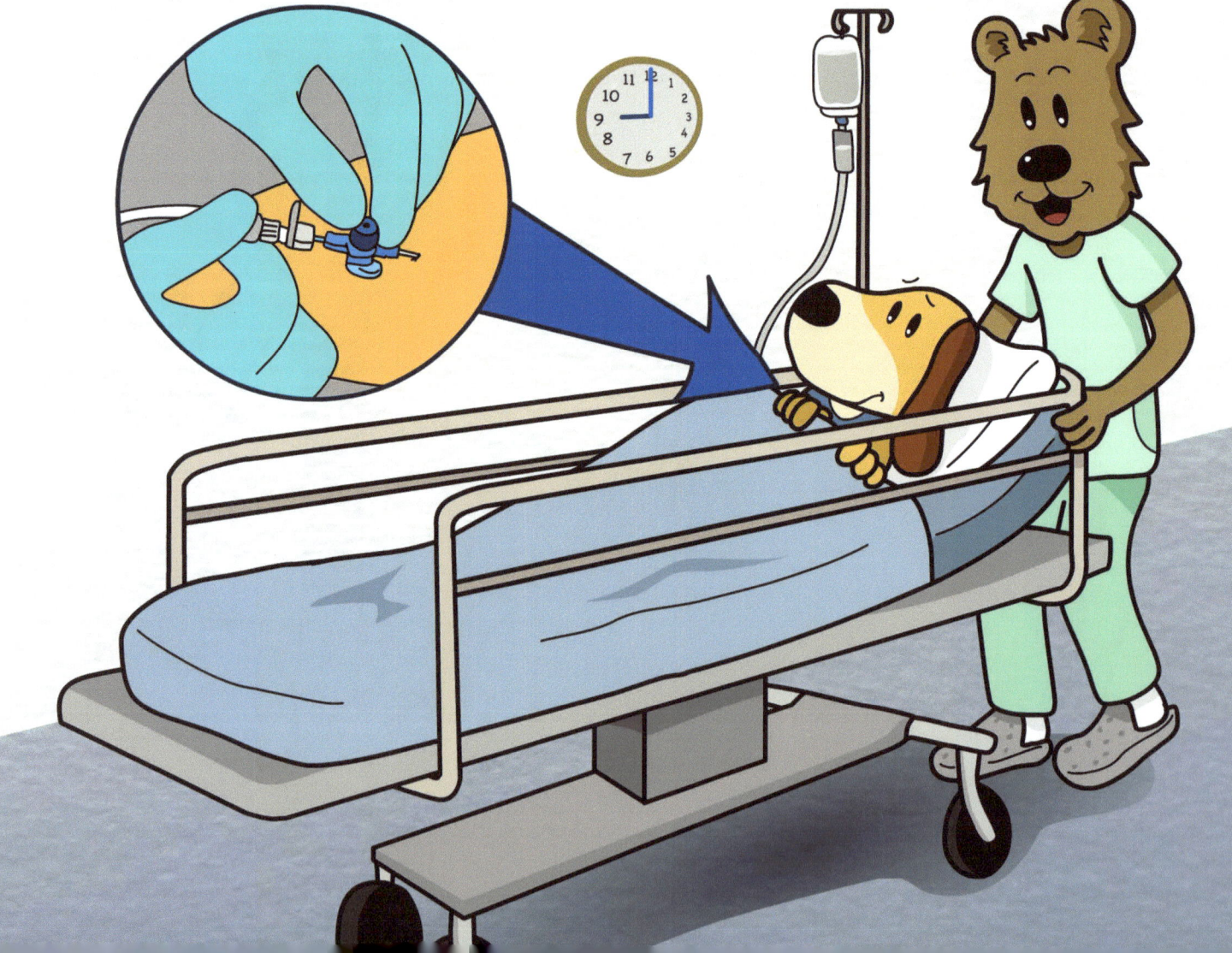

In the operating room, there was lots of equipment and several people dressed in blue and green.

Nurse Rodney helped Sandborn onto the special table where the operation would take place. They placed a pillow under his head and covered him with a blanket. Then the surgeon came in.

"Hi, Sandborn - I'm Dr. Tso, your surgeon" she said cheerfully. "Dr. Seva has told me all about your tonsils. Just a little snip and you're going to be fine!"

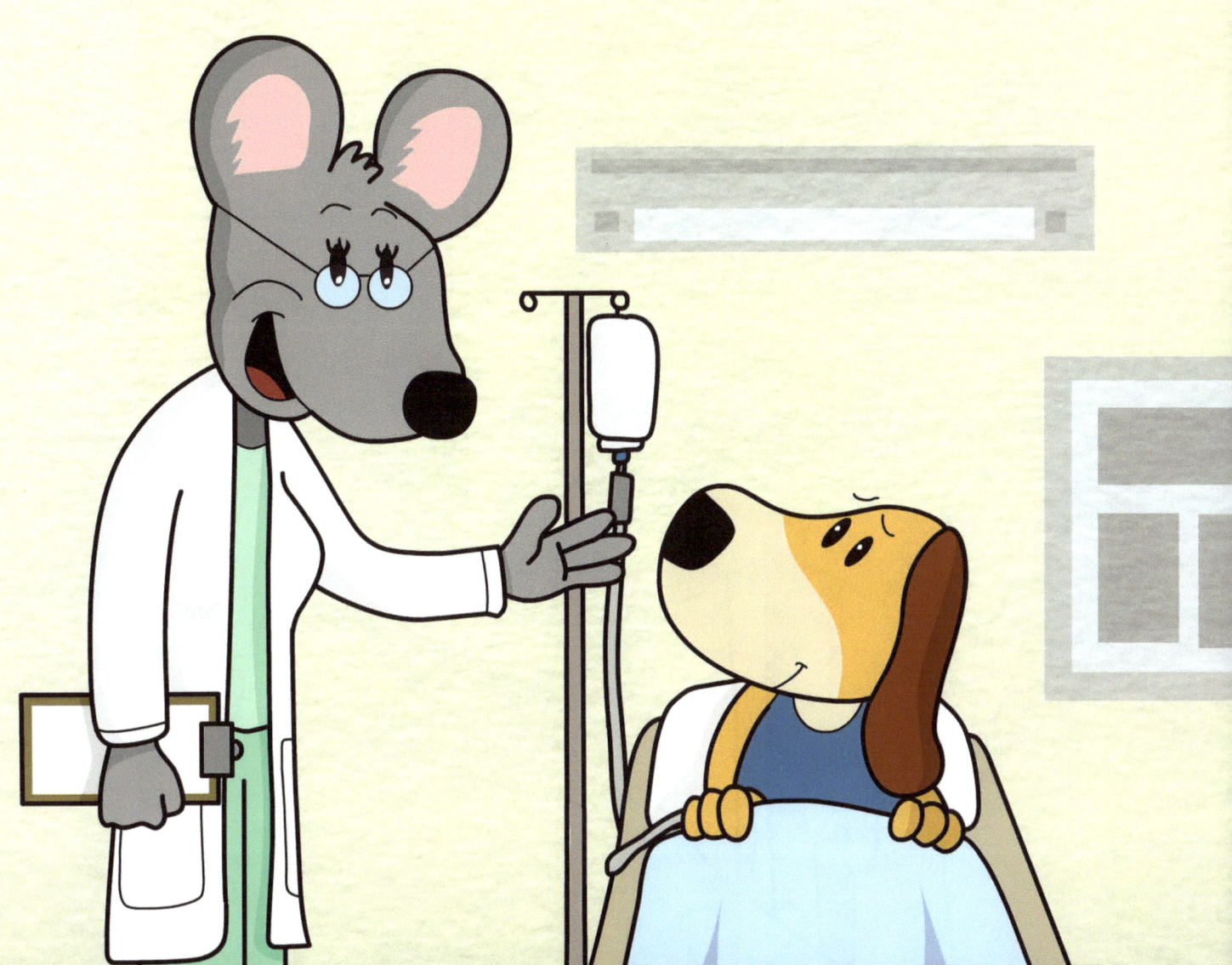

Then, Dr. Yashen appeared to administer the medicine that would put Sandborn to sleep. She also explained that she would use a special machine to help him breathe while he was asleep.
"I will watch over you while you get sleepy and during your entire operation." said Dr. Yashen.

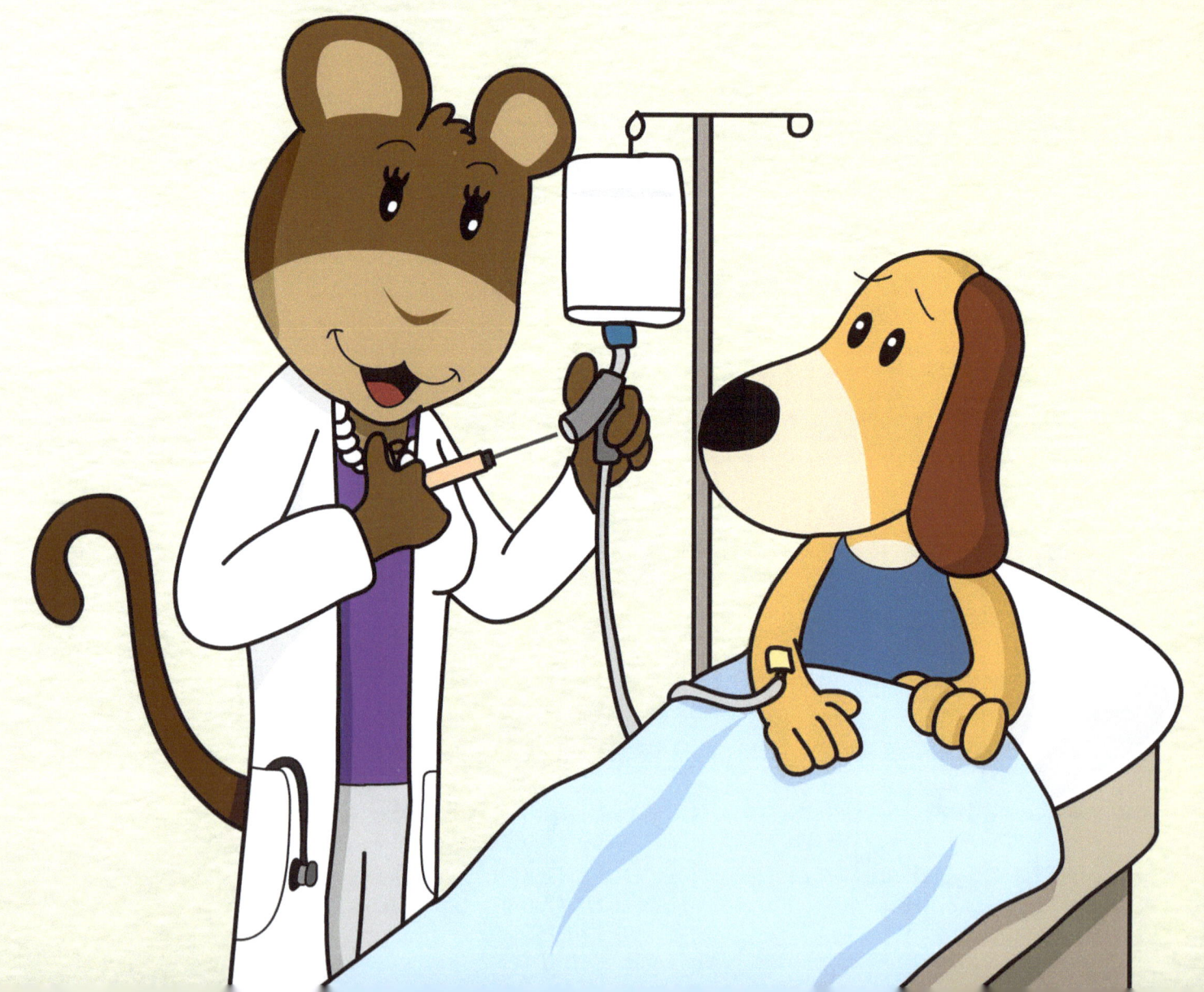

"Are you comfortable?" asked Dr. Yashen. "Yes," said Sandborn.
"Great, now all you have to do is start counting backwards from 100."
"Okay," said Sandborn.
"100, 99..." **Everyone here is so nice.**
"98-97..." **I hope I can have my party tomorrow.**
"96-95..." **Mom is right outside.**

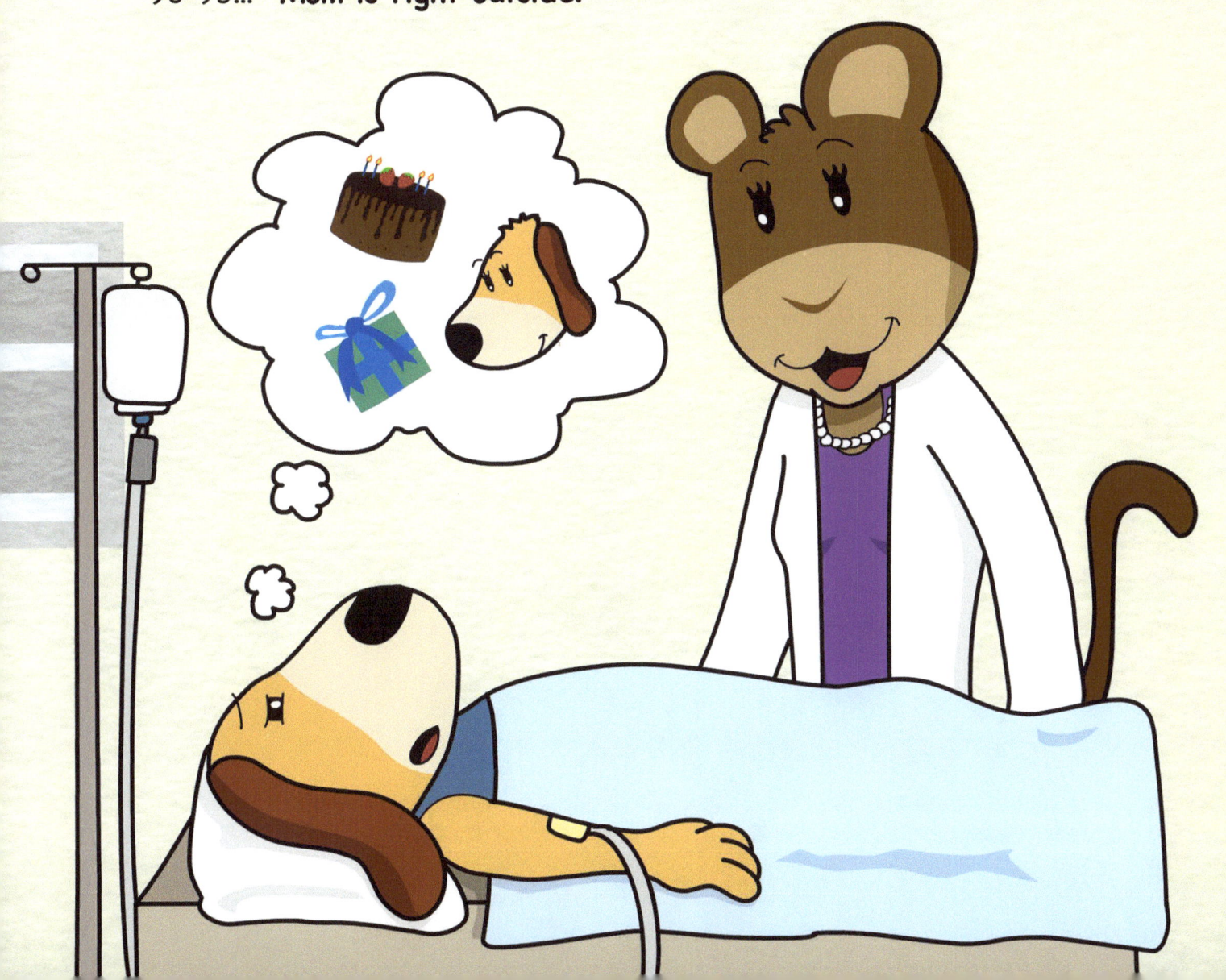

And the next thing Sandborn knew, he was back in his room!

"Hi," said his mom.

"Hi," said Sandborn. "Is it over?"

"Yes, and you did very well!"

But Sandborn felt so thirsty!

"May I have some water, please?" he said.

"Of course," said his mom, bringing him the cup and helping him drink. "Take small sips," she said. And sure enough, as Sandborn swallowed he felt the soreness in his throat that Dr. Seva said would be there after the operation. It would take a week or so to go away.

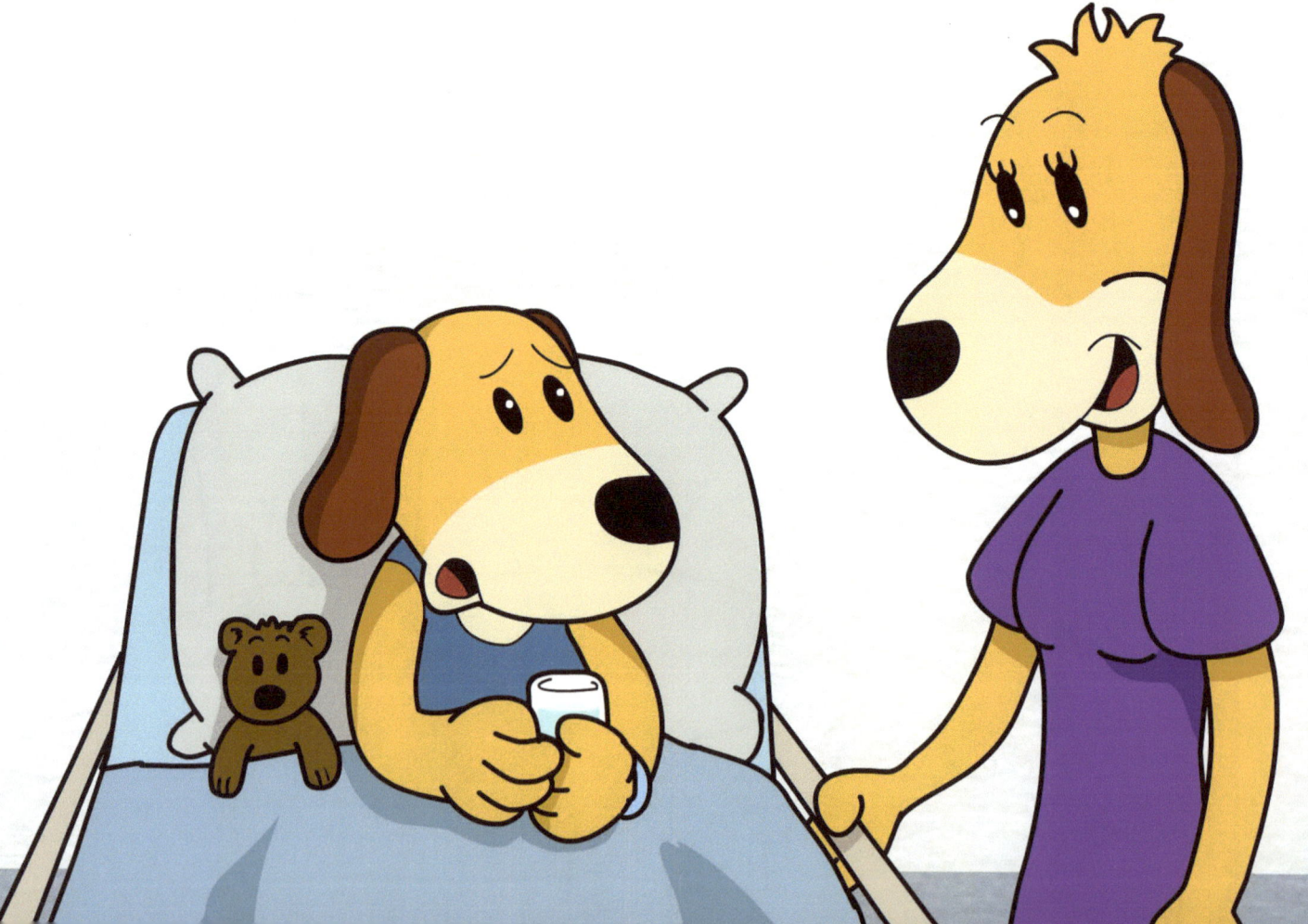

"What about the ice cream?" said Sandborn, breaking into a little smile.
"Oh, that's right here," said his mom with a laugh, going over to a little refrigerator that was in the room and taking out a cup of vanilla ice cream. "Do you want some now?"
Sandborn tried to sit up higher in the bed.
"Mom," he said, "I haven't had anything to eat since last night!"
And they both laughed as Sandborn began to dig into his ice cream.

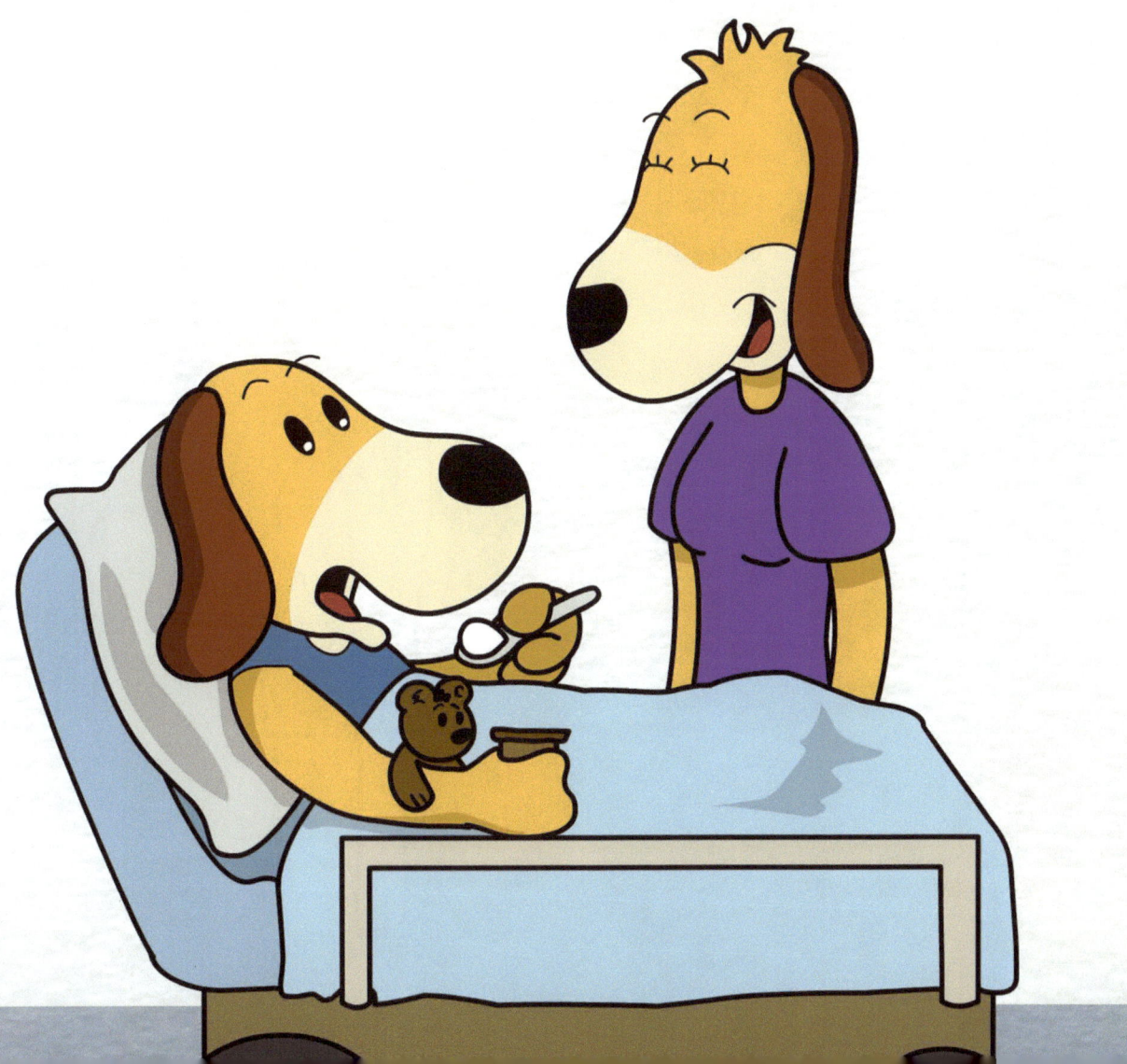

Throughout the day Sandborn and his mom watched TV and played games. Several hospital people came by to check on him-including Dr. Tso, who examined him and said he was doing fine, except for a little fever that she wanted to watch. Dr. Seva, too, came by and said that Sandborn would probably be going home on Sunday, once the fever was gone.

Sunday! thought Sandborn. **That for sure means no party tomorrow!** He felt very proud to have gone through the operation so bravely, but sad that his birthday party wasn't going to take place.

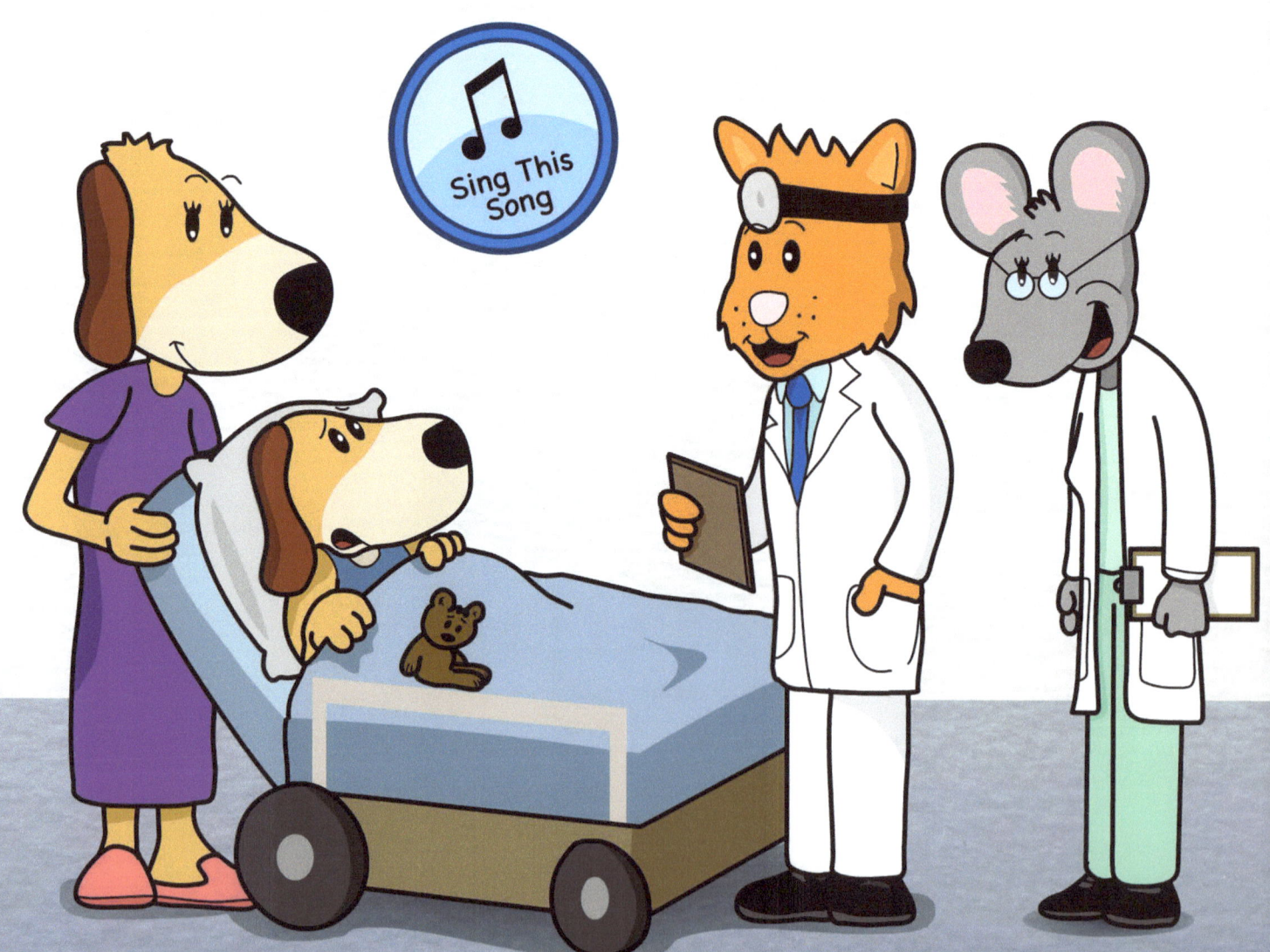

Sing This Song

On Saturday morning, Sandborn woke up early. His mom was already awake.
"Hi, mom."
"Morning, sweetie. How are you feeling?"
"Well, by throat is better than yesterday, but it still hurts and I am very tired. I guess Dr. Seva was right about not sending me home until Sunday."
Breakfast was delivered - creamy oatmeal and applesauce - and for the next few hours Sandborn and his mom watched TV and played games.

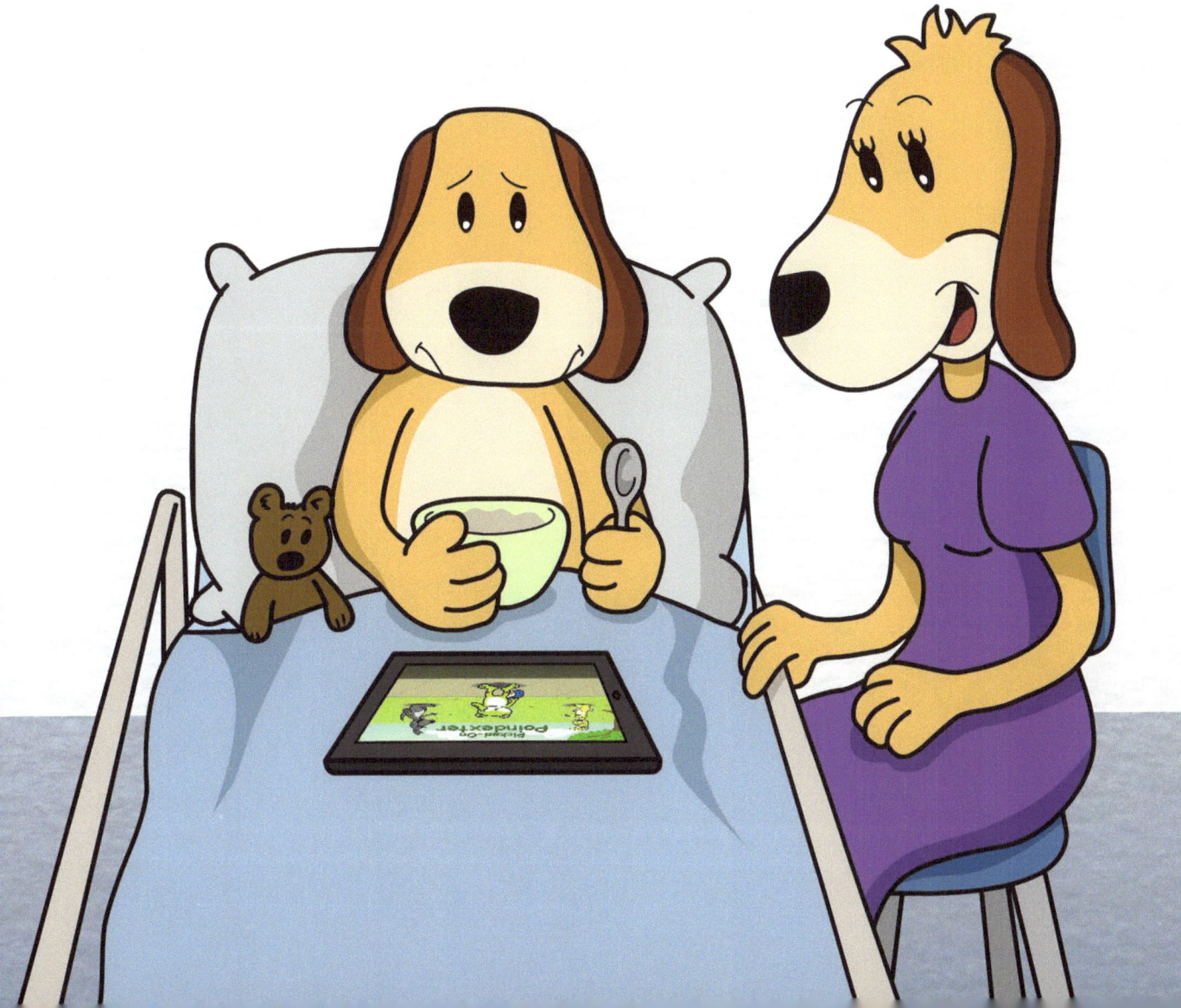

Then, late in the afternoon, Sandborn's mom got a phone call, and stepped out into the hallway to talk. When she returned, just a minute later, she had a huge smile on her face -- and the next thing Sandborn knew, there were voices at the door of his room. "**Surprise!**"

It was Bonky, Poindexter, and Drysdale—and they were all smiling as brightly as could be. They had brought Sandborn's birthday party to him!

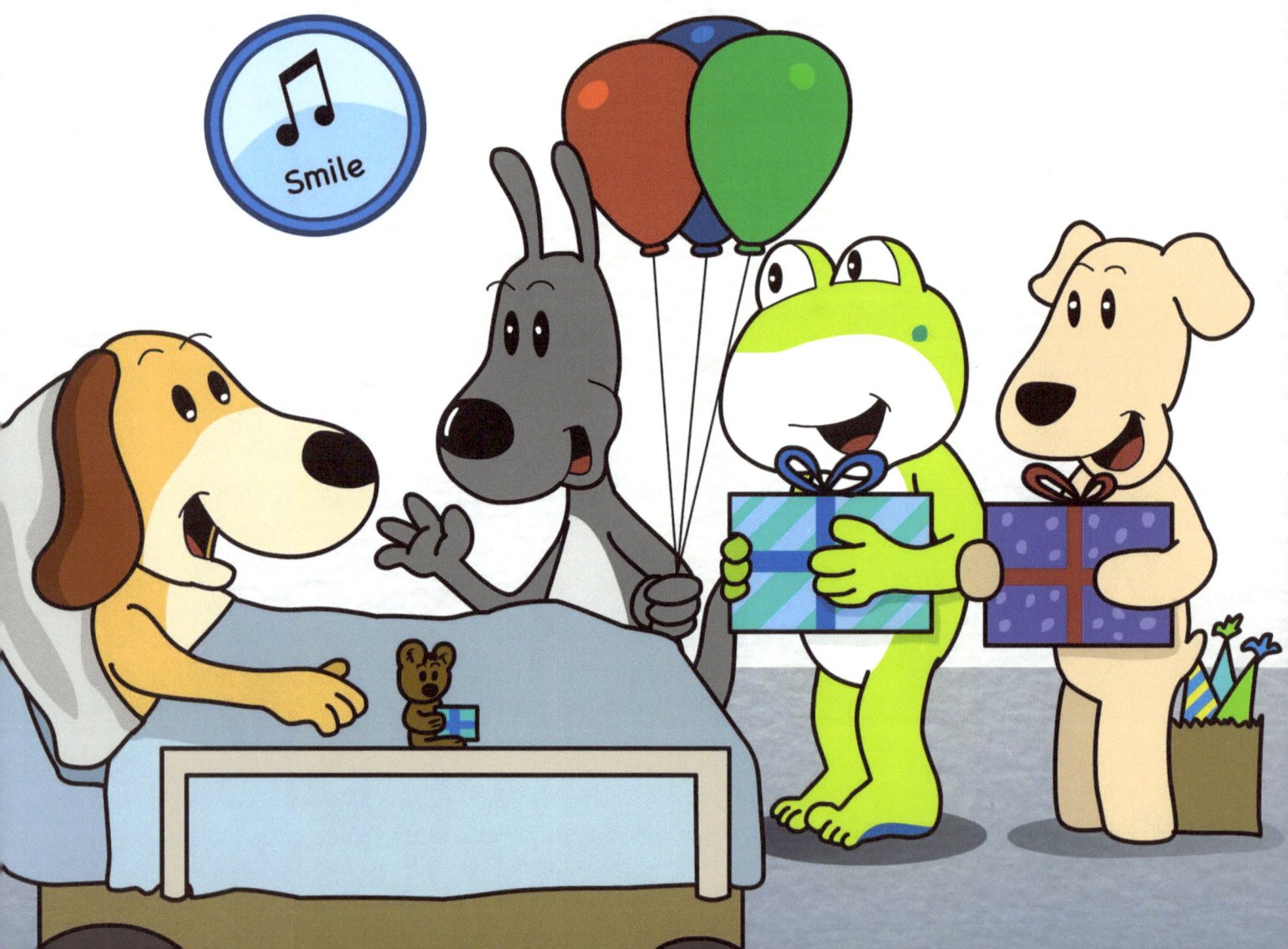

"We'll have a real birthday party when you come home, but we wanted to celebrate with you today!" said Bonky.

"Your mom said it was OK," said Poindexter.

"You guys are the best," said Sandborn, as his friends reached into a bag they brought and took out some party hats, which they all put on.

"Happy birthday, sweetie," said Sandborn's mom.

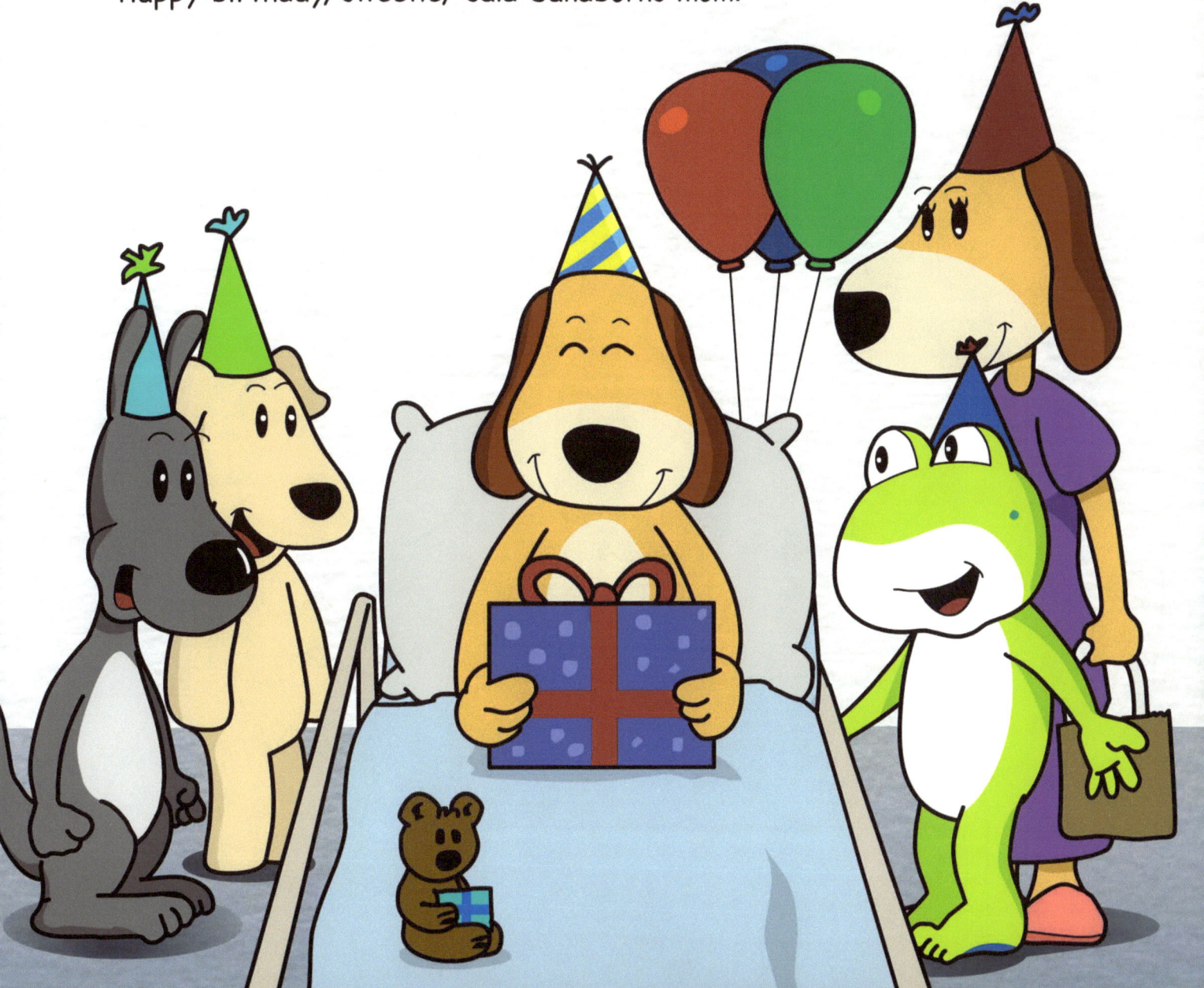

"We have a few presents for you-- games and stuff," said Bonky, "so you won't get bored while you're in bed."
"I brought you a book," said Drysdale.
"Also this," said Poindexter, taking a pint of ice cream out of the bag.
"You said your mom was going to make a chocolate-strawberry cake. So until your real party, how about some chocolate-strawberry ice cream?"
"Yay," said Sandborn, "more ice cream!" This is the nicest birthday ever, he thought.

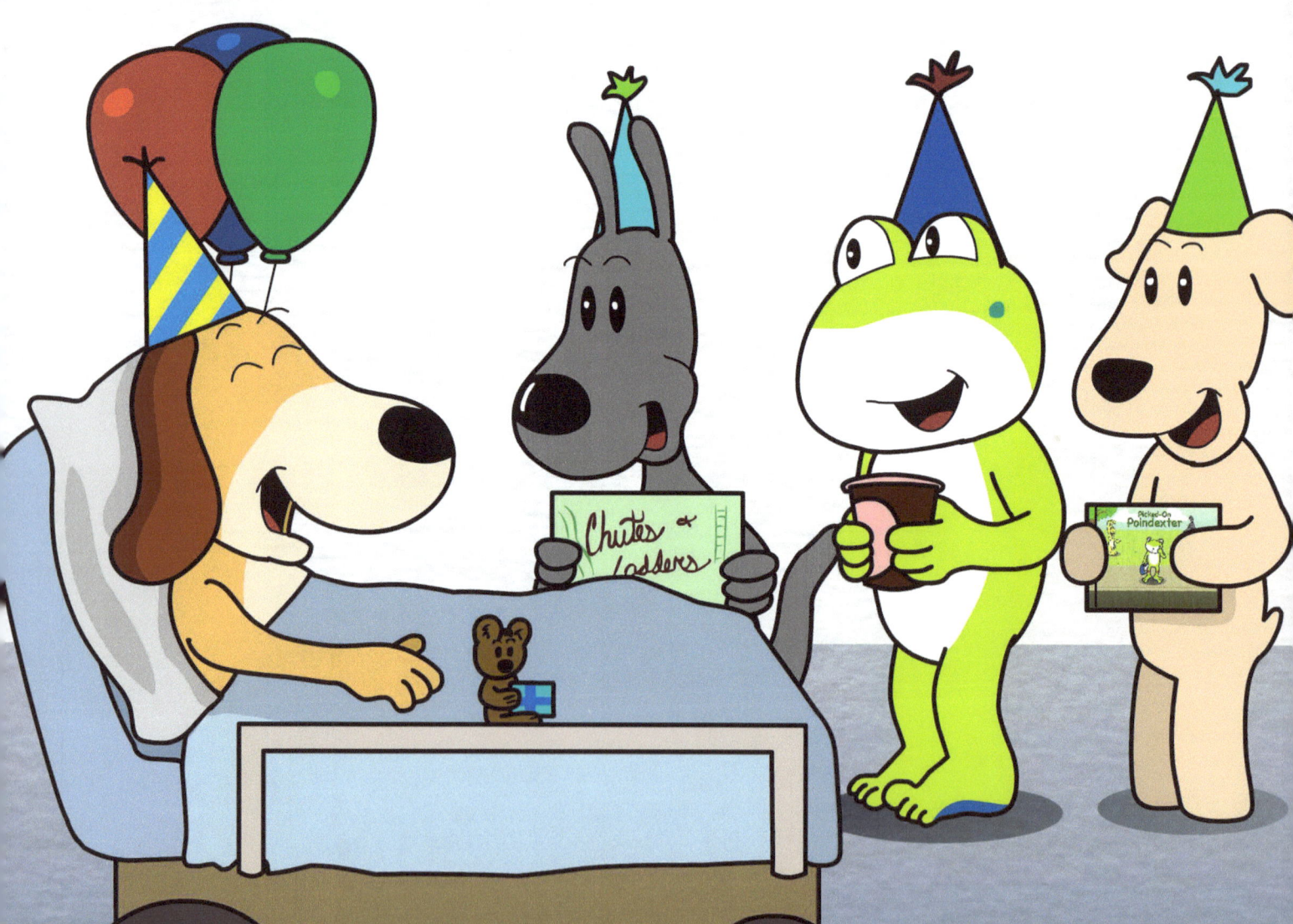

Even Nurse Rodney had some ice cream, when he stopped in to check on Sandborn. And later, as Bonky, Poindexter, and Drysdale were leaving, they promised to help Sandborn plan his real birthday party, which they all decided, with the help of Sandborn's mom, would take place as soon as Sandborn was back on his feet. "Two birthday parties instead of one," he said. "Gee - having an operation wasn't so bad, after all!"

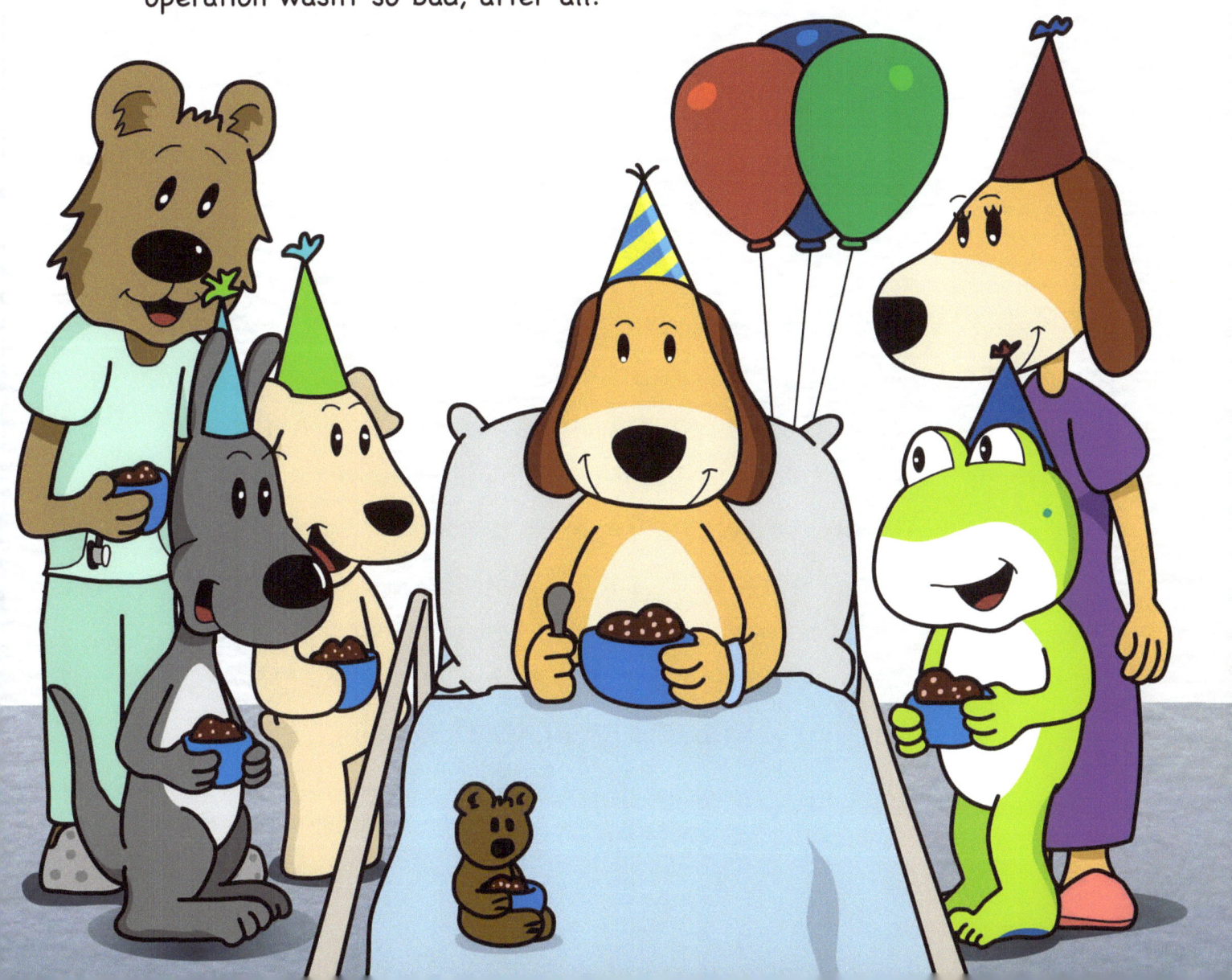

Sniffly Nose

When you wake up with a sniffly nose,
There are things you can do
From your head to your toes.
Things to feel better, things to forget,
Let's try to be silly, and not so upset!
Rub your tummy, clap your hands, and wiggle your toes,
Raise your arms in the air, touch the tip of your nose,
You can stick out your tongue, or whistle a tune,
Give me a hug, you'll feel better real soon!
When you wake up with a sniffly nose,
There are things you can do
From your head to your toes.
Things to feel better, things to forget,
Let's try to be silly, and not so upset!

Feeling Down and Out

I know you're feeling down and out, at times you get upset,
Know I am here for you to squeeze, to help you forget!
So put your worries in a bag, a pillowcase or cup,
Then, throw them out the window and do not give up!
It's hard when you don't feel so well, to keep a smiling face,
But, I will be a cheerful pup if you don't give up!
I know you're feeling down and out, at times you get upset,
Know I am here for you to squeeze, to help you forget.

Sickly

When you're feeling sickly, not so very giggly,
You'll get better quickly when you take your medicine.
When you're feeling icky, oh so very sicky,
You'll get better quickly when you take your medicine!
I'll be back to school real soon,
In my fav-rite classroom.
Being sick will not last long,
'Cause I will soon be strong!
When you're feeling sickly, not so very giggly,
You'll get better quickly when you take your medicine.
When you're feeling icky, oh so very sickly,
You'll get better quickly when you take your medicine!

Sing This Song

Every day can be so long, when you have a little wrong,
Take some time to sing this song, it's a special one for you.
Now the day is almost done, It was not so very long,
'Cause I found something fun to do, I'm singing this song!
La-d, da-d, da-d, da da,
La-d, da-d, da-d, laaa,
La-d, da-d, da-d, da-de da,
La-d, da-da-daaaa,
La-d, da-d, da-d, da-d da
La-d, da-d, da-d deeeee.
La-d,da-d, da-d, da-d-la,
Lad-d-da, da, deee!
Every day can be so long, when you have a little wrong,
Take some time to sing this song, it's a special one for you.
Now the day is almost done, It was not so very long,
'Cause I found something fun to do, I'm singing this song.

Smile

I learned how to change, a sad into a glad,
It's easy to forget, that I was ever sad.
What did I do, to change a sad into a glad?
I put a smile on my face, the best idea I've had!
Smile, Smile, Smile, Smile, Smile, Smile, Smile
Smile, Smile, Smile, Smile, Smile, Smile, Smile!
I learned how to change, a sad into a glad,
It's easy to forget, that I was ever sad.
What did I do, to change a sad into a glad?
I put a smile on my face...the best idea I've had!